JUL - - 2013

## DATE DUE

| AUG 2 1 2013 | | DISCARD |
|---|---|---|
| NOV 0 9 2013 | | |
| | | |
| | | |
| | | |
| | | |
| | | |
| | | |
| | | |
| | | |
| | | |
| | | |
| | | |
| | | |
| | | |
| | | |
| | | |
| | | |
| | | PRINTED IN U.S.A. |
| | | |

# THE
# PALEO
# COACH

Expert advice for extraordinary health, sustainable fat loss, and an incredible body

## BY JASON SEIB

Victory Belt Publishing Inc.
Las Vegas

First Published in 2013 by Victory Belt Publishing Inc.

ISBN 13: 978-1-936608-47-8

The information included in this book is for educational purposes only. It is not intended nor implied to be a substitute for professional medical advice. The reader should always consult his or her healthcare provider to determine the appropriateness of the information for their own situation or if they have any questions regarding a medical condition or treatment plan. Reading the information in this book does not create a physician-patient relationship.

Printed in the USA
RRD 02-13

" Let Jason Seib be *the* Paleo coach in your life to help you cut to the chase and get to the meat of the matter about becoming as optimally healthy as you can possibly be! His nuanced understanding of how to live like our hunter-gatherer ancestors in today's world of iPads, the Internet, and *American Idol* is sorely needed. Other Paleo books may promise to help you lose X amount of weight in two weeks, but *The Paleo Coach* offers you much, much more. Jason realizes that it takes a dedicated commitment to implement a lifestyle change and homes in on key principles aimed at delivering big changes in your weight, health, and outlook on life. "

**Jimmy Moore**
*Livin' La Vida Low-Carb Blog and Podcast*

" *The Paleo Coach* is not just another Paleo book—it's a priceless tool that is absolutely essential for anyone striving to live the best life possible. The insight, advice, and lessons in this book could come only from someone like Jason, who has spent serious time deep in the trenches of the health-and-fitness industry. With his hands-on experience, understanding, and innumerable success stories, Jason reveals what it takes to look beyond the hype and focus on what really matters: your own personal path to health. Everyone should have a coach, and now everyone can. *The Paleo Coach* will change your life. Guaranteed. "

**Sarah Fragoso**
author of the national bestseller *Everyday Paleo*

# TABLE OF CONTENTS

# THINK

# EAT

# MOVE

# FOREWORD
## by Sarah Fragoso

Hi! My name is Sarah Fragoso, national best-selling author of *Everyday Paleo* and the *Everyday Paleo Family Cookbook*. I met Jason at his gym two years ago when I was invited to present an Everyday Paleo nutrition workshop to his clients. Afterward, Jason and I had dinner together, and I got to know a little more about this phenomenal trainer who decided to make his home in northern Oregon, hidden away from the limelight that could be his to enjoy, busily and confidently running his own extremely successful gym.

I learned immediately that what matters to Jason is helping people and knowing that he can. Seeing his clients practically crawl through the doors of his gym for the first time, sick and tired and unhealthy, and months later bound through them, vibrant and healthy and living full lives that they never thought possible. That's the only reward he cares about. Celebrity-trainer status? Meh.

Jason embodies a true passion that I rarely see anymore. Thanks to the misinformation that is force-fed to the masses by popular and unrealistic media circus acts like *The Biggest Loser*, most of us envision trainers as boot camp drill sergeants who admonish you to eat less and move more and bark at you to not give up. This one-size-fits-all, tough-no-love approach never works long term—for anyone. Every single day, Jason's goal is to help folks find their own path to health, and he is relentless in his quest to find the best answer and plan of action to fit the individual needs of each of his clients.

Today, I am truly blessed to call Jason my business partner and friend, and I am writing this foreword because I am confident that this book will help you. Let me rephrase that: I know without a shadow of a doubt that this book will be the stepping stone you need to gain a better understanding of who you are, how you tick, how to get healthy, and, most importantly, how to stay that way!

Why *The Paleo Coach*? Never in the history of the world has an NFL team made it to the Super Bowl without a competent and experienced coach. The world-famous gymnast Nadia Comaneci did not score those practically unheard-of perfect 10s all by herself: Her amazing coach Béla Károlyi was always by her side. World-class boxers? All have great coaches. Basketball superstars? Coached. I think you get the picture. These athletes may have been blessed with the genes to succeed, but without the guidance of a professional who knew what to do with those genes they might have never carried a trophy home, never made the front page of a newspaper.

Why should your own physical challenges be any different? When faced with trying to figure out how your body is supposed to work and why it isn't working, seek professional guidance. If you simply want to live the best and healthiest life possible and obtain your lifelong goals, find a professional who can help you. Think of *The Paleo Coach* as a specialized playbook, complete with all the sneaky maneuvers you'll need to circumvent the obstacles you will inevitably encounter on your journey to health. There are too many books written by "professionals" who gleaned all their information from textbooks or research articles. Only by working for years in the trenches with real people can someone claim the credentials of being a true coach. Jason is that person.

So how will this book help you? This book does explain what Paleo is and why it works and the basic science and principles of the lifestyle from Jason's perspective, but thank goodness it is not just another Paleo book. Jason is the tough kind of coach who makes you sit down fast and listen. He's the loving kind of coach who knows how to say exactly what you need to hear when you need to hear it. Jason will take you to the place where you start to get the feeling that it's all coming together and that you are finally one step closer to figuring this Paleo thing out—and with a rush of excitement you'll realize that it just might actually work!

Jason pours his heart and soul into his message. His strongest desire is to make sure that when you put this book down you will have the confidence to take on the Paleo challenge, that you will understand why this lifestyle is the answer you've been searching for, and that you will revel in the power you have to be the healthiest and most vibrant person you can be.

So now it's time for you to meet Jason and take in all he has to offer. I can't wait to hear your victory yell when you finish the final chapter, as the crowd cheers loudly and you hold high over your head the coach who helped you achieve all you can achieve—your very own Paleo Coach!

# ACKNOWLEDGMENTS

Sitting down to write each day was the only part of the creation of this book that I did alone. Everything I learned and experienced in order to fill these pages required the support of these wonderful people:

Sheryl, Liesel, Capri, and Daphne. Without you, there is no reason for me to get out of bed in the morning. Your support and patience made this book happen. I love you with all my heart.

Kris. My best friend and business partner. Every aspect of my career is tied to you in some way. I can't count the times I called you for help or asked your opinions as I wrote this thing. You have never not been there when I needed you. Not once. I am eternally grateful.

Sarah and John. You are quite literally the reason for *The Paleo Coach*. You didn't even ask me to write it; you told me that I must. Thank you so much for your never-ending support. You both mean the world to me.

Jeromie. You helped me find more research papers, listened to more of my brainstorming, and helped me talk out more crazy notions than anyone will ever know. Please know that I deeply appreciate all of it.

Deb, Angela, Katie, Mike, Erika, Tim, Elane, Debbie, and Jen. Thank you so much for letting me share your experiences with the world. I know it wasn't easy to talk about your journeys, but you gave of yourselves with the hope that your stories might help others. You are all amazing, and I am fortunate to be able to call you my friends.

Robb Wolf. You are my unwitting mentor. I have learned more from you than from anyone else, and I am grateful to you for blazing the Paleo trail. You have always graciously answered every question I have ever asked. Keep leading, and I will keep following.

Mom and Dad. I could tell you that I was planning to build a ladder to the moon, and you would believe in me and support me. Thanks. I love you.

Erich, Michele, and everyone else at Victory Belt Publishing. Thank you for helping me make my lifelong dream come true.

The Clackamas Physical Conditioning trainers and members. You are my foundation, my frontline support, and the best cheerleaders anyone could ever ask for. Thank you.

The Everyday Paleo Lifestyle and Fitness community. Your stories, questions, trials, and tribulations are behind so much of the content of this book, and I truly appreciate the opportunities you have given me to grow as a coach. Thank you for always believing in me.

# THE PALEO LIFESTYLE
## *at a glance*

## Foods to Enjoy
- Meat
- Vegetables
- Fruit

## Exercise
- Walk
- Lift Heavy Things
- Sprint
- Get Flexible
- High-Intensity Interval Training

## Foods to Avoid
- Grains
- Legumes
- Vegetable Oils
- Refined Sugar
- High-Fructose Corn Syrup
- Artificial Sweeteners and Sugar Substitutes
- Soy
- Most Dairy

- Avoid Traditional Cardio

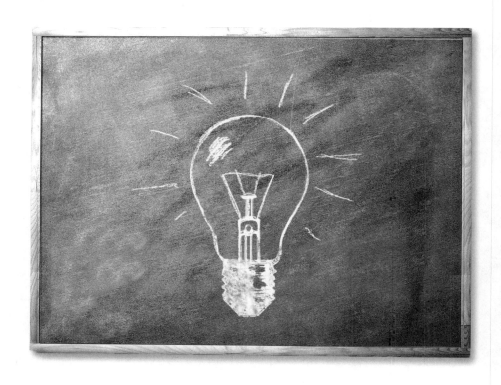

THINK

# INTRODUCTION

## *perspective is everything*

If you cannot see a problem for what it really is, how can you expect to find its solution? Nutrition and fitness remain mysterious subjects to the masses because we have strayed from the logical concepts that make up their basic tenets and have come to put our faith in ridiculous ideals propagated by unsubstantiated hearsay and myth. But have no fear, I come bearing epiphanies.

This book is, like most other books, a result of personal passion. There is very little on these pages that I have not said out loud from atop my soapbox over the course of my career—or that is being conveyed by the mainstream nutrition and fitness powers that be, a fact that only further fuels my passion. It saddens me that the methods I, and many others like me, have used to help so many people are often literally the polar opposite of what those people come to me believing to be true. It disgusts me that so many "experts" can completely ignore so much good science and literally thousands of shocking anecdotal cases in order to leave the same useless, albeit lucrative, protocols in place. It makes me want to scream when I hear nonsense spewing from the mouths of celebrity doctors and trainers who could not possibly have done a shred of research to substantiate their claims. But it warms my heart every time I open someone's eyes to the truth in terms of their health and fitness. That is why I wrote this book, which is nothing more than my best effort to help you see things differently, to show you how to effectively reach and maintain your health and fitness goals. If I am successful, you will be absolutely astonished by what your body will become.

Please understand that I honestly want to help. I think this will become clear as you read on, but I want to mention it now because there is a good chance that you may dislike some of the things that must be said. Most people in the Western world have forgotten what it means to be healthy, and it may not be easy or comfortable to get rid of the notions and habits that don't serve that goal, but it does neither of us any good if I simply hand you a set of nutrition and fitness rules and then whip out my pom-poms and cheer for you like other gurus who never got you anywhere near your goals. No, my mind is made up. I'm going to tell you the truth, even if I make a few enemies. My experience has taught me a lot about who fails and who succeeds, and I intend to share this knowledge with you. Some of these truths may sting a little, but we are going there anyway—there is no other option.

There is not one single trick or gimmick in this book. Not one shortcut. Tricks and gimmicks are for people who are satisfied with short-term, unsustainable results. Shortcuts are fantastic if you want to lose and regain the same ten or twenty pounds over and over and over again. Tricks that cheat the process are an easy sell, but I can't, in good conscience, offer you anything but methods that yield real, lasting results. When we are done here you will see shortcuts for what they really are and always be able to spot their flawed logic in the future.

Paleo nutrition is a powerful life-changer, especially when paired with exercise founded on the same concepts, but it is merely a map from point A to point B. In the end, it will be up to you to decide whether to follow the path as it unfolds before you, and you will do so based in large part upon your understanding of the big picture. If this book is your first introduction to Paleo, fasten your seat belt—this is going to be an eye-opening adventure. If you are a seasoned Paleo pro, I intend for you to exit this ride with a deeper understanding of what you may have thought was nothing more than a diet.

I am not going to rehash every shred of scientific data pertinent to Paleo nutrition and exercise. Robb Wolf did a better job of that than I ever could with his most excellent book *The Paleo Solution*. I will, however, give you everything you need to succeed, and more importantly, make sure you don't have any valid reasons to fail. All the tools and step-by-step instructions are included, but they will not be enough if you don't know what your obstacles are before you come up against them.

Our first order of business is to remove the major obstacles from your path; then we will define Paleo and learn how it should be applied. We will do this by, you guessed it, changing your perspective. Just so we are clear, I'll say it again: Perspective is everything. Let's get started, shall we?

# CHAPTER 1

# the real rules
# of the game

## The Aesthetic Goal Conundrum

I will not try to convince you or anyone else to give up on looking good. I don't believe we will ever change social pressures, and to think otherwise is a pipe dream. But I firmly believe that your perspective holds the key to your success or failure. I know that statement must make me sound like a Zen master chanting "Become one with your body," but give me a chance to explain. Natural selection has shaped us and given us some ground rules. Ignoring what has made us human is a grave mistake. Unfortunately, we often stray furthest from nature's intentions when our goals are based solely on changing the way our bodies look.

In the animal world, nearly everyone is attracted to displays of good genes. Take, for example, this male peacock's vibrant and beautiful tail.

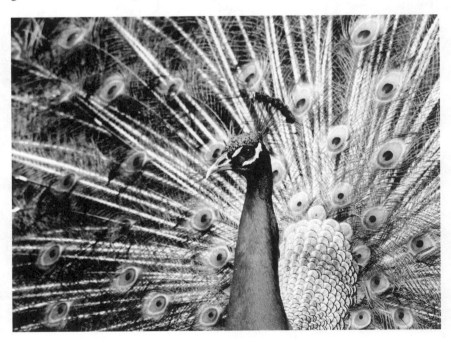

He is not saying, "Check out my dazzling tail! Don't you want to mate with me?" He is actually saying, "Look at the enormous biological expense I can afford. It requires a ton of biochemical energy just to grow this thing. I have to spend valuable foraging time keeping it preened and looking nice, and it weighs me down when I have to escape predators, but here I am strutting my stuff in front of you. Clearly my genes are superior to those of the other males, and your offspring will fare very well if you mate with me." This is an example of the handicap principle of sexual selection, and it basically explains how the best genes tend to win contests for mates, even when elaborate displays are involved that might otherwise attract a mate through beauty alone.

We do not employ the handicap principle, but physical attraction in humans, as in most animals, is also a display of good genes. As long as we are talking about aesthetics alone, we are drawn to bodies that display physical and reproductive fitness whether we like it or not. To put this another way, we are attracted to healthy, fit, capable bodies. You can test this concept for yourself if you don't believe me: ask someone nearby to close her eyes and picture the most physically attractive body she can imagine. Add to these instructions that she must be as shallow as possible and not pick anyone who is endeared to her or more attractive due to any character or personality traits. Once you have given your subject ample time to conjure up some lust, ask her if she pictured an unhealthy person. The answer will invariably be no. In fact, the person brought to mind will be very physically capable and in excellent health. This is one way our genes manipulate us for the good of our species. We do not consciously decide which physical traits we find attractive; we are innately drawn to healthy, fit bodies because they are most likely to contain the genes that, when combined with our own, will give our children the best advantage.

Our minds are also intricately involved in sexual selection, which explains the evolution of music, art, humor, and all other forms of creativity. Geoffrey Miller, in his fantastic book *The Mating Mind*, explains in detail how our minds became a fitness indicator because intelligence is a valuable asset for survival and thus attractive to potential mates. In this aspect, we have not lost our way in modern times. We still hold others in high regard who are intelligent, creative, charismatic, passionate, compassionate, funny, etc. In fact, these traits can oftentimes far outweigh physical attraction, so much so that the person we choose to be with is not always the one who is the most aesthetically appealing. I am absolutely positive that nobody can refute my last statement, but let's be honest, you are not assessing your personality when you're standing in front of the mirror and your inner voice is taking potshots at your self-esteem. "You're not creative enough!" is not something you yell at yourself, so let's get back to judging the book by its cover, even though our mothers told us not to.

You cannot change your genes, or genotype, but you can certainly affect the expression of your genes, or phenotype. Most of the genes that control the way we look, feel, and perform work like switches that are turned on or off by inputs like the foods we eat and how we use our bodies. Take for example, the Australian Aboriginal gentlemen in the picture below.

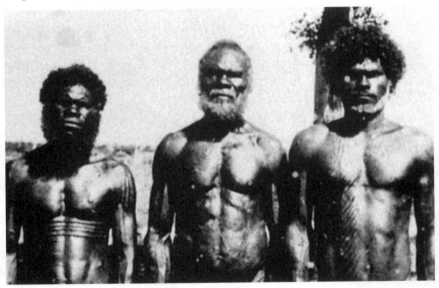

*Indigenous Australians, 1939*

This picture has been passed around the Paleo community as an example of the excellent physical condition of indigenous hunter-gatherers. It suits that purpose quite well, but I would like to use it to make a different point. Australian Aboriginals today suffer rates of type 2 diabetes and heart disease that are among the highest in the world, but at the time this photograph was taken these diseases were virtually nonexistent in these people. Therefore, we can say that they were more genetically predisposed to type 2 diabetes and heart disease than most other populations because the introduction of the same Western foods and unnaturally high carbohydrate diet made them sicker than almost everyone else. Their genetic predisposition did not, however, cause them any problems to speak of before they threw the switch on those genes through the input of "modern" foods.

The same logic applies to your own aesthetics. The current state of your body is mostly a result of the choices you made in the past and how those choices have affected your health. For example, a genetic predisposition to obesity is extremely uncommon, but it is possible. So, yes, I just said that your over-fatted or under-muscled condition is a result of your own decisions and technically your fault, but I am going to cut you (us) some slack, because we have had so much misinformation crammed down our throats by the "experts" and others who would profit from our misinformedness that it's no wonder you haven't been able to escape the typical unhealthy fate of Westerners. (The excuse of ignorance remained in play until you picked up this book and began arming yourself with the truth. But knowledge is power, and so you will be, from this point forward, held fully responsible for your decisions—and health.)

Now for some good news. If we understand that our genes do not prescribe an unavoidable fate, the next step is to admit that we, in large part, hold the reins on our health and physical attractiveness and should therefore stop acting like helpless victims flailing in front of the mirror. However, we must embrace our new, broader definition of the aesthetically appealing body and chuck the ridiculous old one. Our inability to understand that physical attractiveness is an expression of health has led us to lose our minds to such an extent that logic and reason have been almost completely abandoned. See if you can follow this: Fat is undesirable; the opposite of fat is skinny; skinny is therefore desirable. (As a reference, see the tragedy of the *New York Times* bestseller *Skinny Bitch*, by Rory Freedman and Kim Barnouin.) To reveal the silliness in this logic, we need only return to the exercise in which you asked someone to visualize an attractive body. If you are a woman who did that exercise with a man, ask him to describe the body he imagined. I will stake my reputation as a man on the fact that he will not use the words "skinny," "thin," or even "small" in his description. If you are a man, please explain this concept to the next woman who will listen. The story is similar when we flip the genders. Men tend to believe that women love muscle-bound behemoths, when in reality women are also drawn to healthy bodies first and foremost. Attractiveness does not denote size, it denotes health, and health cannot be measured by size alone. There are healthy, attractive bodies that are small, and there are healthy, attractive bodies that are large. In other words, not all attractive bodies are small, and not all small bodies are attractive, but bodies that stay attractive for a lifetime are healthy bodies, so attempting to get smaller without getting healthier does not make sense. It makes much more sense to get as healthy as possible on purpose while you get hot by accident.

Any plan to achieve better aesthetics that ignores health is a trick or gimmick and will probably fail in the long run, if not in the short term. I do not use the words "trick" and "gimmick" to mean an idea someone is trying to sell you on that he knows will not work, although it is possible. I simply mean plans that try to pull a fast one on your physiology and biochemistry. For example, you would probably not assume that the fast track to *peak health* is to restrict yourself to consuming 1,200 calories per day, but this is an all too common way of trying to *lose weight*. Starvation is not normally associated with sustainable sexiness, but it is associated with temporary weight loss, which brings me to my next point.

## Yo-Yo Dieting and Caloric Restriction

I find it quite disconcerting that "yo-yo dieting" is actually a term recognized by most of the Western world. How can we have come to a place where gaining and losing the same ten or twenty pounds more times than we can count is so common that it has a name? I always find it a bit odd when people tell me about how they lost a bunch of weight on some completely unnatural diet and consider it to have been a major success even though they gained all the weight back. When probed they will tell me that they felt great about how they looked but that they were starving all the time, or depressed, or couldn't sleep, or didn't have any energy, or had any number of other symptoms indicating a decrease in overall health and vitality. How on earth can this possibly make sense to so many people? Let's remember the golden rule of aesthetic goals: *Any sustainable improvement in physical attractiveness will be achieved through improved health.*

An often overlooked side effect of yo-yo dieting is loss of muscle mass. When calories are dramatically reduced, cortisol (our primary stress hormone) is released and muscle is catabolized, or dismantled, so the proteins can be used to make glucose (blood sugar). The numbers on the scale may be getting smaller, but it is *weight* that is being lost and not just fat. This seems like a good thing to the dieter who has been programmed to believe that the scale is the ultimate judge of attractiveness. The problem is that muscle mass is precious and hard earned. If you want to be really healthy and live as long as you can, muscle mass is an important part of the equation. Unfortunately, when calories are eventually increased, a stressed-out body will pack on as much fat as possible, mostly around the midsection, to brace itself for the next stress event. Without the stimulus of resistance training, muscle mass does not return. With the next round of yo-yo dieting you rinse and repeat, further decreasing the ratio of muscle mass to stored fat until you are eventually a squishy mess at your original weight or heavier. Good times.

To make matters worse, our bodies are excellent at adaptation, and lots of yo-yo dieting will eventually cause your body to believe that the constant ebb and flow of stress events is the norm, and fat loss will get even harder as the body deems stored fat more valuable and holds on tight. All that temporary success followed by miserable failure is also quite hard on the old self-esteem. How many times can you try really hard, only to fall flat on your face, before you begin to assume that you are just too weak to reach your goals? Since everyone *knows* this is how to achieve weight loss, you are not likely to think, "Wait a minute—something just doesn't seem right here."

The authors of an observation study titled "Multiple Types of Dieting Prospectively Predict Weight Gain During the Freshman Year of College" came to some conclusions that you might find interesting. Here is the abstract (bolding mine):

*The freshman year of college is a period of heightened risk for weight gain. This study examined measures of restrained eating, disinhibition, and emotional eating as predictors of weight gain during the freshman year. Using Lowe's multi-factorial model of dieting, it also examined three different types of dieting as predictors of weight gain. Sixty-nine females were assessed at three points during the school year. Weight gain during the freshman year averaged 2.1 kg. None of the traditional self-report measures of restraint, disinhibition, or emotional eating were predictive of weight gain. However, **both a history of weight loss dieting and weight suppression (discrepancy between highest weight ever and current weight) predicted greater weight gain**, and these effects appeared to be largely independent of one another. **Individuals*** *who said they were currently dieting to lose weight gained twice as much (5.0 kg) as former dieters (2.5 kg) and three times as much as never dieters (1.6 kg), but the import of this finding was unclear because there was only a small number of current dieters (N = 7). Overall the results indicate that specific subtypes of dieting predict weight gain during the freshman year better than more global measures of restraint or overeating.*

According to this study, the women who were the most likely to gain weight were those who were actually dieting when the study began, and the women who were most likely to gain the most weight were those who had dieted the most often in the past and/or those who had lost the most weight in the past. To rephrase that, trying many times to lose weight through caloric restriction appears to be a good way to become heavier.

OK, so yo-yo dieting is definitely not the answer because it does not work, and it does not make sense that all indigenous hunter-gatherers, all humans pre-agricultural revolution, and all the animals on the planet are miserable and starving and better at being miserable and starving than you are.

Am I telling you to be happy with an overweight body? Of course not. That, too, would be nothing more than a pipe dream. I am simply making the point that the path to better health leads to a hot body by accident, while the direct route of the purely aesthetic goal often ends in frustration. Why is it necessary to pursue health first in order to look good? Now we are getting into the good stuff.

## Why Aesthetic Goals Are Bankrupt

Time for an observation or two of my own. These are purely anecdotal (loosely backed by observation studies like the one I mentioned a moment ago), but I believe most quality trainers with years of experience and success will back me up here.

Throughout my career there has been one consistent indication that a client will most likely struggle to achieve her goals: the unwavering attachment to purely aesthetic goals with no regard for improving health. When it comes to goals and motivations, everyone who walks into my gym can be placed in one of two groups. The vast majority hate their bodies, or at least some part of it, and are desperate to change themselves and find some relief from the torment of their own disapproval. The small minority love their bodies enough to know they deserve better. This type of person usually finds success very quickly and without a lot of stress. Unfortunately, the first group includes at least nine out of ten people, and if those people do not have a radical shift in self-perception they tend to further divide into two sub-groups: those who never fully reach their goals but convince themselves that halfway is good enough, and those who are just passing through and will be leaving the gym soon. Why would the purely aesthetic goal be the bane of success for so many people? Other than the fact that directly pursuing only visible results skips the necessary step of improving health, I am not 100 percent sure, but I have a couple of theories.

First of all, I have long suspected that the type of person who spends a lot of time worrying about how he looks might also be the type of person who worries more about everything. If so, then we can assume he will have elevated cortisol levels, which means more fat and less muscle. If you are a stress case with way too much on your plate and bad sleep habits, major physical changes will be a huge challenge. Throw in some stress about your appearance and you are officially stuck in a negative-feedback loop: Worrying about how you look = more stress = more cortisol = more fat/less muscle = more worrying about how you look.

Second, body loathing probably goes hand in hand with low self-esteem in most cases. Whether the relationship between how you look and how you value yourself is correlated or causal, the outcome is often difficulty with compliance. An attitude of "I don't deserve better than this" will block your path to success every time it rears its ugly head. If you sometimes feel that efforts to improve yourself are pointless, especially if you have struggled with your self-image for a long time, you will probably cheat on your diet and skip workouts more often than you should. This, of course, also creates a negative feedback loop. Cheating = more self-loathing = more feelings of hopelessness = more cheating.

Third, desperation can sometimes make us do crazy things that end up being counterproductive. For example, walking might help a person lose a few pounds and feel good. This might then lead to the assumption that running is even better, which results in full-blown cardio. Traditional cardio, like distance running, as opposed to walking or sprinting, tends to be perceived by the body as stress, which increases cortisol, thus breaking down more muscle and storing more fat. In other words, fat loss gets really tough unless most of your muscle mass is emaciated first. Here's another example: While a small reduction in calories is not necessarily a bad thing and will probably aid weight loss, desperate minds often take this concept to such ridiculous extremes that regaining any lost weight is inevitable, which usually results in more desperation. Even at a gym like mine, where we provide an accurate road map to health and fitness, this more-is-better mentality gets the better of people and robs them of the results they deserve. When this happens, they rarely assume it was because they stopped looking at the map. Since more *must* be better, they honestly believe that they went above and beyond the call of duty and still failed. This is another harsh blow to an already pummeled sense of self-esteem.

Paleo nutrition and responsible exercise are certainly important, but the "how" pales in comparison to the "why" for most people. In other words, you might be given 50 well-researched scientific papers and 100 examples of anecdotal situations in which people used that information and achieved remarkable results, but these things will never be able to compete with what happens in your head when you get up in the morning, step on the scale, and pick apart your body in front of the mirror. You are not likely to accidentally stumble on a body you love if your head is not in the right place. You can, however, accidentally end up with a great body, but you will need to love it enough to get it healthy first.

Besides the need to get healthy, there is one more reason you must stop hating your body if you ever want to reach your goals.

## You Can't Fix a Body You Hate

In all my experience, with all types of people, at nearly every possible fitness level, I have yet to see anyone turn a body she hates into a body she loves. To be honest, I don't think it can be done. Sure, bodies can be changed in remarkable ways, but the minds that hate them just get more critical. In other words, you need to change your perspective to appreciate and celebrate your gains. Keep hating your body and your successes will be overlooked while you abuse your self-esteem with thoughts like, "I still have so far to go!" or "Yeah, my hips look better, but my thighs are awful!"

If you have been on a thousand diets, continually lose the same ten or twenty pounds, weigh yourself at least once a day, can't look at yourself naked without disdain, and absolutely loathe shopping for clothes, you probably will not win this battle without some serious soul-searching. Don't get me wrong, you can certainly build a body that crushes others with envy, but you probably won't see it. You already know people who are exactly what you might become. They have bodies that you would kill for, and yet they are insecure about every inch of themselves.

Of course, this is an extreme example, but any amount of this behavior saddens me. It is so frustrating as a trainer to watch someone make unbelievable gains only to nitpick her body under a magnifying glass while the rest of the world admires her success in awe. I have seen as much as forty pounds of fat lost in only a few months go seemingly unnoticed by the person doing the losing. I have seen the success of clients inspire the new people in my gym, yet I have to walk on eggshells when I talk about their goals lest I bring them to tears. I have seen bodies evolve into absolute magnificence and remain covered virtually head to toe on hot summer days. What is the point of all this? Why go to all the trouble of busting your butt in the gym and eating right if your mindset makes your goals unattainable?

I believe that this might be how some people develop exercise addictions. Insecurities that run deeper than skin level are addressed by changing the body, instead of changing the head. When this strategy proves futile, as it will, the assumption is that more exercise must be the answer. If food is blamed for low self-esteem, the result might be decades of yo-yo dieting or a more serious eating disorder.

Let me be clear: Dissatisfaction with the way you look is not a crime, and I am not telling you to settle into the idea of being overweight or out of shape, but I would like you to stop and think about your motives and whether or not your head is in the right place to acknowledge success when it comes.

## How Pam Got Her Head Right

Pam is a member of Everyday Paleo Lifestyle and Fitness, an online fitness-and-nutrition coaching community that I co-founded, and an awesome person. She posted the following on the EPLifeFit forums in May 2012 in a thread titled "Getting My Head Right!"

*I have been struggling mentally and emotionally lately. My struggles have really had nothing to do with the nuts and bolts of Paleo. I still feel like when it comes to the food, exercise and other Paleo lifestyle factors I'm still living in the zen of Paleo. Except for my body image. I started hating the reflection in the mirror. I started seeing every physical flaw, all the loose skin, all the old stretch marks, and honestly perceiving myself as much larger than I actually am. I was really down in the dumps about this ... frustrated and angry, both at my current physical state and my old obese self. I got really frustrated that I haven't and may not hit my original goal weight from when I started losing weight (only 10 lbs away). I know none of these things SHOULD matter, but they started to matter to me ... actually, they all became a big eff'ing deal to me.*

*I was watching the finale of* The Biggest Loser *the other night and was totally struck by a comment from Cassandra, one of the eliminated contestants. She talked about being in the fitting room recently trying on her first ever bikini. She expected the experience to be a negative one, but it wasn't. She ended up saying,* **"In all my imperfect glory, I just love myself so completely."** *The girl could not stop BEAMING the entire time she was on stage (and she stood there during the weigh-ins of a number of the other eliminated contestants as she held top spot for the consolation prize for a while). I can't help but imagine that she's got some of the same physical "scars" from obesity as I do. And there she was, talking about loving herself completely in all her imperfect glory ... not in spite of all the imperfections.*

*I realized I had my head all wrong. I was blind to all the glory and beauty in my imperfections. That saggy, loose belly? It's a sign of how far I've come and how much I've changed. I lost sight of that and let my inner critic bring me down. I was so blinded that when I put on size 6 pants last weekend and they fit perfectly in the dressing room my first thought wasn't "WOW, way to go me!" but rather "I would probably be in a smaller size if it wasn't for this loose skin." How messed up is that?*

*I think the switch is flipped. I want to be kinder to myself and start living in the present rather than the past. I want to find the positives everywhere in my life instead of giving any headspace to the negatives. I'm doing things now that I never thought I could do and I want to keep challenging myself and growing rather than living in fear and on the sidelines like I used to. Instead of looking at my saggy arms in the mirror, I'm going to start treating myself to my own little gun show.*

*I'm not there yet, but I think I'm now back from that negative space and starting out on the right track to getting to the point of loving myself in all my imperfect glory.*

*Where did this all come from? I truly think that the 21-day totally clean eating really allowed me to feel these feelings and emotions more strongly than I have in the past when I've been under the power of food. Taking away the emotional power of food in my life and improving my mental clarity let all these thoughts and feelings come through loud and clear. In the spirit of being kind to myself, I don't regret the thoughts and feelings. I needed to hear and feel those things to come out stronger on the other side.*

What a beautiful example. To this day, Pam continues to make improvements, but as you can see from her post, she almost missed them. If she had remained focused on all the wrong things, never seeing the huge strides she was making, how long do you think she could have kept going? With a positive perspective, Pam is able to celebrate each little step in the right direction while also appreciating how far she has come overall. It's good to be Pam!

# CHAPTER 2

## playing for the right reasons

### What Is Riding on This?

It's time for another test. If your primary goal is to change the way you look, I would like you to do the following exercise without skipping ahead. I honestly believe it will be great for your perspective.

1. Imagine, if you will, that I take my magic wand out of its charger, reach through the pages of this book, and—*poof!*—make you look exactly the way you do in your dreams.

2. Set this book down and take your perfect body to a pen and paper and make an exhaustive list of all the things that have been miraculously improved in your life by your new physical appearance. Remember, we are only talking about your appearance here. You cannot list things like "I have more energy" or "I am a better softball player." Do not pick this book back up until you have made your list.

3. Now go back over your list and put a checkmark next to each item that is not completely based on your own opinion of yourself.

Do you have any checkmarks? Are you sure? You might need to scratch some off your list. For example, you cannot put a checkmark next to "I am more confident," because your lack of confidence is a decision *you* are making based on how *you* feel about your appearance. You might legitimately be more confident if you feel more attractive, but we need the word "feel" to make this statement true. There is not a scientifically measurable point of fitness below which everyone suddenly becomes insecure. You know people whose physiques do not fit the mainstream "hot body" description, but they are confident nonetheless. Also, you have had days when you were not comfortable in the clothes you were wearing and no compliment anyone could ever pay you would change your mind. Confidence, or lack thereof, is not constant across all people of a certain size or shape because we each decide when to allow our self-image to negatively affect our confidence.

In all the times I have asked clients to participate in this exercise I have never seen an example of an improvement to appearance solving anything but self-imposed problems. I believe the valid checkmark is a myth. I once had a client tell me that if she improved the way she looked her boyfriend would quit telling her she was fat. Her opinion of herself was to blame because if she loved and respected herself, she would have ran the jerk out the door the first time he popped off his idiot mouth. We choose whose words hold value for us, and people who love themselves do not allow bitter, unsupportive, hurtful fools to hold sway over them.

It is also important to acknowledge what is real and what you may be fabricating. Let's say you walk into a room in which there are ten people you have never met. If you are not comfortable in your skin, you probably take a quick, maybe subconscious, survey and rank yourself among the strangers. If you made the assumption that you are near the bottom of the pack, or worse, that everyone in the room looks better than you and disapproves of the way you look, you will have taken a pretty serious blow to your self-worth. Nobody wants to feel as if they are the least attractive person in any group. But do you have any tangible reason for jumping to such conclusions? Nope. Nobody ever yells out your place in the pecking order when you enter the room. So, in this particular situation, you have quite effectively beaten yourself into submission, and now you have to deal with these negative feelings for the rest of the day.

OK, OK, I admit that your emotions are your emotions and I would be naïve indeed if my message were entirely based on a "suck it up and love yourself" mantra. Don't worry, there is more to my plan, but it is important that we rationalize this stuff before we move on.

Here comes some of that tough love I warned you about back in the introduction. If the things you say to yourself inside your head are unsubstantiated in real life, you probably cannot come to a place where you will be happy with your body. To put this another way, if you tell yourself things about the way you look and who you are that are not actually grounded in anything real, like the opinions of the people who care about you, then *you* are the biggest obstacle in your path. *What if your self-deprecation is the only thing keeping you from succeeding? How many of your day-to-day frustrations are based entirely and exclusively on your own opinion of yourself?* These questions need answers, and they need them now. We have other things to attend to, but there is no point in moving forward if you are going to continue to stand in your own way.

If you need to do some soul-searching, have at it. This book does not have an expiration date. It will not self-destruct if not read in thirty days or less. When you are ready, we are going to take a look at some incredible changes in perspective and the priceless rewards they render.

# Angela

Angela is a remarkable person and I am grateful to know her. She had been a member of my gym for months when I asked her to meet me for coffee to talk about sharing her story for this book. However, I had no idea just how amazing her story would be. I did not want to simply present you with another success story and a set of before-and-after pictures like you have already seen associated with countless diets in books and on the Internet. The message is always the same– "Look at the amazing results these people got when they did The _____ Diet!" That is just marketing and it isn't really helpful to you for anything but motivation. Angela's story, on the other hand, is a slow evolution that took her from a place of frustration and pain to a new perspective, a new body, and a new lease on life. I would like to take credit for all Angela has accomplished, but her revelations were mostly her own and what I added was no more than icing on the cake. Each of us has taken a different path to get to where we are now, but I think we can all relate to Angela's journey on some level. It is my hope that you might stand on her shoulders and glean something from her hard-earned epiphanies without having to work as hard as she did. Let's start at the beginning.

Angela's mother was always heavy, but she believed gaining weight was simply what happened after you had kids, and she didn't really let it get her down. Her father was active and never more than twenty or thirty pounds overweight. Angela received plenty of love and support from her mom and dad, and I could hear her love for them when she told me her story. She doesn't blame her parents for her own tumultuous battle with her weight. Her mother never even made the common mom mistake of passing on her own insecurities with comments like, "Sweetie, you just have the Jones butt" or, "You have the Smith legs, and they will always be big. Get used to it." As she got older, Angela picked up on subtle clues that her mom may have been a little uncomfortable with her weight, but there was no glaringly obvious body loathing being transmitted from parent to child in her family.

"Growing up, we had Ding Dongs and Twinkies and stuff like that in the house," Angela said. "But we always had family dinner, and Mom would make all the food from scratch. She put a lot of emphasis on cooking at home, but we were still surrounded by all these other junk foods that were also considered normal and part of every day." Unfortunately, this actually sounds like an average American household to me, and certainly very much like the one I grew up in.

It is, of course, likely that Angela subconsciously learned more from her mother than she realizes, but her situation was not one in which she was abused, or told she was fat, or put on diet pills when she was twelve. "Actually, my mom used to tell me I'd be beautiful if I wore a burlap sack and it didn't matter what I looked like on the outside, beauty was on the inside, and I really believed that," she said. "I still believe it to this day, but it was a big eye-opener when I realized that everybody else didn't think that way. They judge you solely on your outward appearance and *then* they would get to know you."

When Angela was in the seventh grade, the style for the girls was to wear leotards with shorts over them. "I'd gotten that outfit for the first time and I was nervous to wear it because you had to have just the right figure," she said. "I thought I could pass, but when I wore it to school, one of the boys in the hallway actually told me I should not have worn that outfit. Right there it was like, 'Wow, people notice how I look and it's so important that they are actually going to mention it to me.' And so that was a kind of a turning point for me, where I became more self-conscious, more aware of how I looked and how other people perceived me. It became really important to me."

According to her doctor, Angela was not overweight. "I guess I was on the heavier side of average," she said. "But I didn't have a cheerleader body so I got teased." By eighth grade, the ruthless teasing she had to endure and the teasing she witnessed other kids being subjected to had already pressured Angela into believing that there was one specific body size and shape that was the ideal, even though it was never overtly acknowledged. I am sure this belief placed her firmly in the majority.

Despite the fact that the ideal-body concept is irrational, most of us buy into it on some level. Most people try to quantify attractiveness. Don't believe me? What sounds more attractive to you, size four or size ten? You picked size four, so now do a quick Internet image search for "size ten models." Did you end up with a lot of pictures of stunningly beautiful women? Of course you did. Compare them with size four models if you like, but you will find no clear winner. This is just another example of how irrational we have become when it comes to attractiveness and aesthetic standards. Attraction is innate. It is the way we have destroyed our ability to think logically about it that is self-destructive and needs fixing. If we really give it some thought, we all know better, but it does not change the fact that Angela's ideal body perspective is all too common. She felt as if the world were telling her she should be ashamed if she didn't look exactly like an ideal that really doesn't exist.

"And that's seriously how I felt," Angela told me. "Like I was broken and I needed to be fixed, but didn't know how. I just felt sort of lost, low self-esteem, low confidence, all that."

It's sad that being a typical kid often means ending up with typical insecurities, so I don't know how this story could have played out any differently. It may have helped if Angela's mother and father knew what you are learning now, and it would be nice if kids weren't horrible to one another, but let's not lose total touch with reality.

The ignorance of early childhood is bliss, but eventually we all reach an age when we begin to place a value on attractiveness, and there is no going back. By the age of fourteen, even compliments held a subtly ominous threat to Angela: "I guess I kind of felt like if I became obese and those compliments stopped, I would lose some part of my self-worth."

It is heartbreaking to think that this young girl had already decided that her self-worth could be distilled down to nothing more than her physical appearance, and that everything else that made her wonderful and unique ranked far below. But to make matters worse, she was slowly beginning to feel as if she were doomed: She was not happy in her skin, but nobody offered her an alternative to what seemed like her inevitable fate of getting heavier.

By age sixteen, Angela was beginning to struggle with depression, and her self-image was largely to blame. Eventually the situation started to get really bad. "It was just basically the common knowledge about food that I was acting on at that time," she said. "So you want to lose weight? Well, you just reduce what you eat, count your calories, and don't eat fat. So I would do that, and it wouldn't work. Then I would take it to the extreme, and I actually became anorexic. I was so proud of myself when I would go a whole day without eating. I was anorexic on and off from age fourteen to sixteen. I never did it for too long—maybe a month on, two or three weeks off—because I feared the negative health consequences and I feared the disappointment my parents would feel if they ever found out. I never wanted to make them think they had somehow failed me."

Angela's beliefs about fat loss at this time are shared by the huge majority of the Western world. In her mind, she was clearly overweight because of the total quantity of food she consumed and her physical appearance was completely unrelated to health. This warped perspective is at the root of all eating disorders. If it were a commonly held belief that physical attraction is a display of good health, and that therefore to get more attractive you should get healthier, nobody would ever starve herself.

Angela never got to the point of becoming emaciated. She didn't have enough willpower to force herself not to eat, and this led to guilt, which led to about a year of intermittent bulimia. "We would go out to dinner and I would eat multiple platefuls of food," she said. "I knew that by the time I got home some of that food would be digested and I would almost feel panicky. I felt like I needed to get home right away so I could throw up. I would eat junk food, too, knowing that I was going to throw it up. So I started making terrible food choices. But bulimia is very difficult to sustain. I just wanted to be able to eat normally, but when I would try, the weight would come back and I would feel even worse about myself."

Thus, the vicious cycle appears to affirm everyone's assumptions about food. Starvation makes you thinner, and thinner is good. But starvation is not sustainable, and eating normally again increases weight. Since being healthy and taking into consideration the types of foods we should eat are not part of the equation, it is easiest to just blame genetics and curse at yourself for being too weak to spend the rest of your life starving. It is very difficult to find a way out of this madness when the feedback seems to make sense: *When I eat more, I get bigger, so caloric restriction is the answer to my misery and woe.*

"It hurt every time I would fail," Angela said. "I would wonder why I couldn't be strong enough to do what everyone else was able to do." The assumption here was that either the thinner girls were better at starving themselves or they were lucky and didn't need to. This comes back to a misunderstanding of genotype and phenotype. Remember the Australian Aboriginals and their modern struggle with type 2 diabetes and heart disease? The same rules apply here. Angela's genes may have made it more likely for her to gain fat than you or I would if we all ate the same modern foods, but if none of us ever ate those foods we would never know who was predisposed to what. Of course, when the whole world is on board with the same misinformation, it is not likely that a sixteen-year-old high school student will come to the conclusion that everyone is eating incorrectly and that she is just suffering a little more for it than those she envies.

At this point in Angela's story she begins to take the first of many small steps in the right direction. When I asked her how she escaped bulimia, she said, "I was miserable and I knew it wasn't something that I could sustain long-term. I'm kind of a planner by nature, and I didn't want to be bulimic for the rest of my life."

The next step was to start blaming a macronutrient, specifically fat. Angela didn't jump from one fad diet to the next, but she yo-yo dieted nonetheless. She estimates that she gained twenty to thirty pounds during her freshman year of college, despite adding cardio to her weight-loss regimen. When she was nineteen, Angela took a job at her local university, where the work environment was very stressful. Shortly thereafter she received a diagnosis of depression and irritable-bowel syndrome, but to her absolute delight the medication she was prescribed caused weight loss. She said, "I was nineteen years old, I weighed 138 pounds, and I was actually comfortable in my own skin."

Hurray? Not so fast. Situations like this often make matters worse. Angela was taking a drug, complete with side effects, prescribed to her because her doctor found it easier to treat her symptoms than to look for the cause of her imbalance. Which part of this is healthy and sustainable? That's right, none of it. The cause of her excess fat was certainly not a deficiency of antidepressants. In fact, the cause of her *depression* was also not a deficiency of antidepressants. Nobody gets depressed because her Prozac gland is damaged. All Angela had experienced was a masking of problems that still lurked in the background and would eventually return to center stage if not addressed. Unfortunately, when you do not know what causes your problems and how to fix them, these brief and unsustainable moments when things seem right are really only setting you up for the next failure and all the psychological bruising that comes with it.

Fortunately for Angela, through all her inner turmoil at the time, she was levelheaded enough to know that she did not want to be medicated. She was soon to be married to Brett, the great guy who is still her husband, and she did not want to walk down the aisle on medication. I think sometimes it is easier for people to hide in the relief they finally find in a drug, despite the fact that they know things are not right. Angela wanted things to be right and she was beginning to question why "right" was so elusive. When I complimented her for thinking so clearly in tough times, she said, "When I look back, I think my life could have really gone in a much worse direction."

After finally quitting her stressful university job, Angela worked at a store that sells running shoes. She said, "This was kind of my first step into a more holistic approach to the body and health. I was around people all day who were trying to lead healthy lives and take care of their bodies."

One day, Angela sold a pair of shoes to a nice man and his wife, and after a fun hour with the couple, the man mentioned that he was a chiropractor. Angela had been suffering from low-back pain since she was fourteen, so she made an appointment to see him. The good doc was able to help her a lot, and they hit it off so well that she ended up working for him. He was great at his job, but Angela said, "More than the chiropractic care, it was his approach to health that really changed my life. Basically, he believed that our health was affected by three aspects of our environment and what we subject our bodies to—chemical stress, emotional stress, and physical stress—and everything we come into contact with in our daily lives can be put under one of those umbrellas. This meant that good health could be found by managing your environment."

Notice the phrases "subject our bodies to" and "managing your environment." These phrases denote responsibility and control. If everything else this man taught her was complete bunk, which it was not, Angela was still learning the basics of some very important lessons. First, her health was determined by inputs. She had made decisions that had resulted in the mess she was in; she did not draw the short straw or forget to rub the Buddha's belly and got stuck with a load of bad luck. Second, she held the reins. If bad decisions got her here, good decisions could get her out.

By age twenty-four, Angela was attending seminars on nutrition and health with her chiropractor boss. She was exposed to a lot of different concepts, and the good doctor taught a nutritional protocol that was very similar to Paleo, but none of it was really sinking in. One particular speaker made note of the fact that our genes have not changed in the last 10,000 years, and the geneticists in attendance were happy to confirm that he was correct. "That was such a novel concept to me," she said. "I was hearing this stuff over and over, and I had been given all these tools to change my health, but I still wasn't doing it."

Through all this, Angela was still suffering from a poor body image, weight fluctuations, and all the frustration and tears that go with that territory. It did not help that her husband, Brett, was one of those guys who stayed lean and well-muscled regardless of what he ate. He always told Angela that she was beautiful, but she felt bad about herself, so she didn't really hear him. She knows better now, but at that time she was sure that Brett was turned off by any excess fat on women. She also knows that she came to this conclusion completely irrationally. On one particular occasion, she asked Brett if he had a problem with her weight gain and he mentioned that he had been with his ex-girlfriend when her weight increased from 119 pounds to 142 pounds and that he had been unfazed. Angela said, "Ten years later I still remember what his ex-girlfriend weighed. And so of course I kept that number in my head back then because I decided that 142 pounds must be the limit."

Since Brett had never mentioned anything about weight gain changing her attractiveness in any way, I asked Angela how she had extrapolated his disapproval from the things he did say. She said, "When we watched movies together I would point out heavy actresses and tell Brett how I did not like the way they looked. I would instigate it and he would agree with me. That is how I gleaned from him where he stood on appearance."

This scenario is all too common. None of us has a detailed dossier containing everyone our spouses, partners, or dates have ever found attractive, nor have most of us ever been told that there is a specific range of attractiveness our significant others deem worthy of their attention. Instead we tease little fragments of information out of them and then manufacture the rest, making sure to create a few unreasonable standards for ourselves along the way. You might consider taking a little time to think about what you actually know to be fact and what you may have filled in yourself. In reality, we have no right to impose these things on anyone. Would you let someone tell you what traits you find attractive? Yeah, neither would I.

At twenty-seven, Angela became pregnant with her daughter and gained eighty pounds. After three years of cardio and a lot of calorie counting, she finally got the baby weight off, but she was back where she started. That is definitely a lot of time and energy spent to get back to a weight she wasn't happy with in the first place. The good news is that her focus was starting to shift away from aesthetics, but her journey was not over yet. "I was done with the misery of obsessing about food and how I looked," she said. "I was trying to change my attitude and accept who I was."

Acceptance is a step in the right direction, and certainly better than self-loathing, but it falls short of happiness because it is basically apathy induced by defeat. When you feel as if you have tried everything, giving up might seem like the only way to salvage your sanity. I completely understand this stage, and I do not fault anyone for going through it, but you have to get moving again. This is not your final stop.

"I was just going to love myself," Angela said, " and when you do that, it's so easy to become complacent. It was a more socially acceptable way of giving up."

Acceptance did not last long because Angela didn't like the way she felt. In the pursuit of more energy, she found herself taking yoga classes, kickboxing classes, and those cardio-with-tiny-dumbbells classes in which light weights are used to get everyone huffing and puffing while a headset-equipped instructor energetically calls out drills for an hour. She stuck to this plan for a couple of years, between the ages of twenty-eight and thirty, and she actually lost some weight, but she was still frustrated. "I kept wondering why I was still carrying around all this chub. I felt like I had so much further to go despite all my hard work. And I didn't like those thoughts in the back of my head telling me I needed to do more cardio every time I ate anything or I would go backward."

The concept of doing cardio to burn more calories than you eat is the other side of the same coin as caloric restriction. You can stress out over eating too much, or you can stress out over trying to expend more calories than you consume, but both are better for losing happiness than losing fat. Angela was no exception and her frustration remained intact.

This is where her story really begins to look up and we start to see just how remarkable Angela truly is. It was around this time that she began to think more and more about her health and she was slowly starting to ask different kinds of questions. The most important of these questions were, "What did people do before they could drive to the grocery store and buy all their food off a shelf?" "What did people eat before all these chronic diseases became a normal part of life?" "People were not always sick, were they?" It is simply amazing to me that she started thinking this way on her own.

"I was searching high and low for someone who had figured this out," Angela said. "Somebody had to know the answers to my questions. This information could not have died with our forefathers." After attending so many health seminars with her chiropractor boss, she knew that there was in fact a time when people did not suffer from the high rate of obesity and noninfectious disease that we do today.

Angela also began to notice that modern medicine is based on treatment. We get sick; doctors treat the sickness. "I started to see this great divide," she said. "There was this symptomatic approach to health care which broke everything down into small parts and tackled them one at a time. But why not just be healthy and get rid of all that crap in one fell swoop? So I started to focus on what makes the body healthy."

With this new concept in mind, Angela took interest in real, unprocessed food. One of her newfound resources was a nearby farm that sold fryer chickens. On one particular trip to the farm, the nice farmer lady asked if she wanted to take the chicken feet, too. Angela was taken aback and asked why she would want chicken feet, but was intrigued when she was told that they were used to make broth. When Angela inquired further, the woman showed her a cookbook called *Nourishing Traditions*, by Sally Fallon.

Sally Fallon is the president and treasurer of the Weston A. Price Foundation, and Dr. Price was a remarkable pioneer. He was a dentist who traveled the world and documented the correlation between nutrition and healthy teeth, which led to his realization that traditional foods begat healthy bodies. He looked at cultures all over the world and kept coming to the same conclusions. When the diet of any culture became overrun with Western foods, the health of those people suffered. His research resulted in dietary guidelines that are very similar to Paleo, and they are light years ahead of the Standard American Diet, but they do not reach far enough back into our evolution, in my opinion. This is not at all to say that the Weston A. Price Foundation has not done a lot of good and helped many people.

With her introduction to Fallon's cookbook, Angela realized that other people really had asked the same questions she had been asking. She said, "Oh my God, I have found the Holy Grail, and it's in this woman's kitchen!" It is amazing how the answers are often so close at hand when we ask the right questions.

In this one moment of relief and elation it is crystal clear that Angela's goals had changed. The years that she spent fretting over her appearance were not driven by a desire to answer questions about human health. What she did not yet know was that she had finally stepped onto the path that would actually allow her to reach those aesthetic goals.

"When I found Weston A. Price I knew I was on the right track," Angela said. "I felt it immediately. But I did not lose weight and I still felt lethargic and fatigued. And then, even on the Weston A. Price protocol, my daughter was diagnosed with leaky gut, she had tooth decay and hair and skin issues. These are not signs of a healthy child. That's when I knew that we were not 100 percent right yet."

Angela kept digging and found some new clues. "I wanted to eliminate grains and sugar," she said. "When I would experiment, going a couple of weeks without either one, I would lose weight and feel better. I would also hear about the success that other people were having with the elimination of those things. But Brett was in love with bread, and he was having a hard time believing grains could be a problem." Brett is not the bad guy here, he just was not convinced yet, and Angela, like most people, had a hard time resisting bad foods when they were so readily accessible.

When she was thirty-one, Angela got pregnant with her second daughter. "A few things ran through my mind at that time," Angela said. "First, I was relieved that I didn't have to deny myself food anymore. We ate according to Weston A. Price nutrition, and although I was figuring out that eating any amount of grains or refined sugars is what made me pack on weight, I thought that limiting my portions would be sufficient. To my disappointment, I still gained seventy-two pounds with that pregnancy. Second, a part of me feared any amount of excess weight gain because it took a ton of effort to lose it the first time. I did not really enjoy the group classes at the big corporate gym, and the thought of having to put in all that work in exercise classes that didn't show great results was not something I was looking forward to."

Angela was still wrestling with the idea that grains and sugar were a big part of her problem, but she was also beginning to realize that exercise would always play an integral role in health. She had not yet come to the conclusion that she did not exercise properly in the past, but fortunately she dreaded those methods anyway. "I told Brett that I could not wait to get back into the gym and start exercising after having my second baby, but I was not excited about going back to yoga and cardio. He would always tell me that I needed to be lifting heavy weights, but I didn't feel like that was my thing."

It just so happens that Brett drove by my gym every day on his way to work. One day he took it upon himself to call me and make an assessment appointment for Angela. To be honest, it was the first time an adult had ever called me on behalf of another adult, and I must admit that my hopes were not very high prior to the appointment. I assumed that Angela would lack motivation since someone else appeared to be pushing her through my door, but I could not have been more wrong.

Brett told her that nutrition was a big part of our program at my gym, but Angela was a little worried. She told him, "If it's anything like the Standard American Diet I'm not going in there! I'm not even stepping one foot in there!"

So, completely by chance, Angela sat down at my desk and heard about Paleo nutrition for the first time, and it turned out to be the missing piece in her puzzle. "It helped that there was a title attached to that kind of eating because it gave me something I could go research." She did not have to go far. I referred her to *The Paleo Solution*, by Robb Wolf, and she also found plenty of helpful blogs and online resources.

I'm not sure what it was, but something I said must have won Brett over. Angela told me, "Driving home from meeting with you, Brett said, 'Let's do it. Let's go Paleo. Let's cut out the grains and sugars and just do it.' I was so happy. We went home and cleaned out the cupboards, throwing away everything that was not Paleo-friendly."

## All the Pieces Come Together

From there, the results came fast. It was as if Angela's body was starving for the inputs she was finally giving it. She gave up on her aesthetic goals, thinking about her weight only as a marker of health, and then she reached those goals by accident. See for yourself.

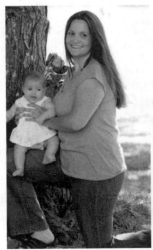
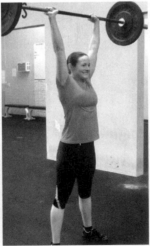

*Here is Angela when she arrived at my gym.*

*And here she is just four and a half months later.*

At the time of our interview, I asked Angela how much weight she had lost, and her answer made me proud. "I actually don't know exactly," she said. "I haven't weighed myself in a while. I got rid of my scale on my sixth-month anniversary in the gym. I kept it around for a while because I knew this was the last time in my life that I was ever going to go through a major weight loss and I was having a blast watching that number go down."

Please don't get hung up on the amount of time it took Angela to make these changes, because in reality she was healing her body little by little for a couple of years before she found my gym and Paleo nutrition. The point of this story is to illustrate the Aesthetic Goal Conundrum. Angela remained frustrated until she changed her focus and set her sights on peak health. Once she had the facts, everything seemed to effortlessly fall into place, and she ended up with results that encompassed the old goals that she had convinced herself were unattainable.

Angela used to see the scale as judge and jury. When she first started exercising properly, she found a whole host of other accomplishments to focus on. Her goals changed and she added many new challenges to her list, but most importantly she was finally having fun doing good things for a body she loved, instead of despising every minute of the torture she endured trying to escape a body she hated. Take a look at what she is capable of now:

Back Squat: 150 lbs.
Shoulder Press: 90 lbs.
Dead Lift: 245 lbs.
Bench Press: 112.5 lbs.
One-Mile Run: 8 min 14 s
Plank Hold: 2 min 15 s
Weighted Chin-up: 10 lbs. (Yes, Angela can do a chin-up with ten pounds of *added* weight!)

If any of these movements are unfamiliar to you, check out YouTube for a basic idea of what they look like. I say "basic" because you may see terrible form, but you will get the idea.

When Angela starved herself and trudged through cardio in the past, the results were less than stellar and all she got was a little smaller. When she changed her perspective and began to pursue health as her primary goal, she got smaller and leaner than she ever had in the past, but the other benefits were myriad.

I called Angela and asked her to compile all the benefits she has experienced since implementing a Paleo lifestyle (eight months and counting at the time of writing), including proper nutrition and exercise. She emailed this list to me the following morning:

- A painful bunion has completely healed.
- Her cellulite is nearly gone. ("There is a little left, but the improvement is huge!")
- Her tooth sensitivities are gone. ("I had a lot of them due to receding gums.")
- Her dandruff is gone.
- The pelvic-floor issues she suffered since the birth of her first child resolved.
- Her hemorrhoids are gone.
- Her attention span and focus are improved.
- Her memory has improved.
- Her psoriasis (mild) is gone.
- Her joint stiffness and aches are gone.
- Her skin color/tone is improved.
- The smoker's wrinkles on her upper lip and her crow's feet are diminished.
- Her heart palpitations are gone.
- She can get up off floor without assistance. ("I used to need a nearby chair, railing, table, etc., to hoist myself up.")
- She can get into and out of cars much more easily.
- She can sit cross-legged on the floor. ("I couldn't sit on the floor for more than ten minutes in any position, but sitting cross-legged for any length of time was impossible.")
- She can sit in a perfect "L" shape on the floor—legs straight out in front of her, spine perpendicular to the floor. ("Before, my upper back and shoulders always rounded and my entire back would hurt.")
- She has much better posture.

- She can pick up her kids without any pain.

- She can carry both kids at the same time without difficulty.

- Her older daughter (forty pounds) can ride on her shoulders during family walks, even on uneven terrain and uphill, with ease (none of which was possible before).

- She can carry her younger daughter (25 pounds) in a baby carrier for hours without any discomfort or pain. ("My shoulders and back used to burn, and the strap would dig into my waist, which was very uncomfortable.")

- Her sinusitis is gone after more than eight years!

- Her feet have arches again after collapsing more than a decade ago.

- Her hands and feet aren't cold all the time.

- There's no more fluid retention in her ankles and lower legs.

- Before Paleo, Angela would experience numbness and weakness in both legs after getting out of a car. There were several occasions when she thought she would have to sit down to avoid collapsing. This has not happened in many months.

- It is much easier for her to get her children in and out of their car seats.

- She has better hand-eye coordination.

- She can confidently take stairs two at a time now. ("I always had a fear of falling on stairs.")

- She can work in her garden without any pain or discomfort from bending over, lifting, hauling, etc.

- She can push and maneuver a heavy wheelbarrow full of compost or sod.

- Shoveling is much easier.

- She can play chase and tag with her daughter. ("I actually *want* to play chase and tag with my daughter!")

- Her knee pain is gone.

- Her overly dry skin is now more moisturized and healthy.

- She looks younger.

- Her nails are stronger.

- Her acne is gone.

- She has better balance and coordination.
- She has quicker reaction time and reflexes.
- Her candida is better ("Give me a couple weeks and I believe I will be able to say it's gone—hooray!").
- Her sweat doesn't smell when she works out. (*I swear I never once noticed an unpleasant odor about her, but she added this to her list so here it is.*)
- She no longer sweats excessively at night.
- She sleeps better and she wakes up feeling more rested and ready to start her day.
- It's also easier for her to wake up. ("I used to be slow to wake up and quite grumpy. I would be downright angry if someone woke me up before I was ready.")
- She has no more bloating or cramping during her monthly cycle.
- Her bruises heal *much* faster. ("It used to take about two months for a minor bruise to go away").
- Her foot pain is gone.
- Her left hip used to "click" every time she took a step, but that has almost completely disappeared.
- She has much more energy. ("A ton more!")
- Her libido is greatly improved.
- Housework is easier. ("I no longer dread it, and I get it done so much quicker. I've noticed that picking up the kids' toys is especially easier, and I'm so much faster at it too. I'm also much more effective at scrubbing the counters, stove, and dishes.")
- She is much less moody. ("I can bounce back right away if something frustrates or upsets me, whereas before I'd struggle to shake negative feelings and sometimes I'd get caught in a downward spiral that I couldn't seem to stop. At times like that I'd say 'I'm in a funk,' and those funks could last a couple days. I'm happy to say that I haven't gone into a funk for many months now.")
- Her anxiety is gone!
- She has a lot more patience when dealing with her children. ("Parenting is fun again.")

44

- She doesn't have negative/depression-like thoughts anymore.
- Her adrenal fatigue is gone.
- Her hypothyroidism is gone.
- Her blood pressure is up to a healthy level. ("My low blood pressure was most likely due to the adrenal fatigue that I had since college.")
- Her hypoglycemia is gone.
- She can kneel on hardwood/ceramic floors without pain.
- She doesn't fret and worry about things the way she used to.
- Walking for long periods is fun instead of tiring. ("And my feet don't hurt afterward, either.")
- She can walk briskly. ("It sounds silly, but I used to *try* to walk at a brisk pace, but I'd hit a wall and no matter how much I willed my body to go faster, I just couldn't do it.")
- Her senses of taste and smell have improved.

**Here are some improvements Angela expected to see that did not quite turn out the way she thought they would.**

**She thought she would have more confidence.** "I do have more confidence," Angela said, "but it's because I know I am physically capable of doing things, like being able to carry multiple bags of groceries and my daughter at the same time without worrying that I may not be strong enough or that I might drop her. As for body-image confidence, I am definitely more comfortable in my own skin."

**She thought she would have greater self-esteem.** "I realize now that I have always had high self-esteem," Angela said. "If I didn't, I would not have thought my life and health were worth improving. Through this journey, I have come to realize just how much I love myself and my body because I have been willing to make huge lifestyle changes in an effort to give my body the best—and it has been greatly rewarding!"

**She thought Brett would be more proud of her.** "I realize now that he has always been proud of me. It was me who was not proud of me."

(Angela also said, "I know this is not about me, but I thought I would add it to the list anyway. Brett has worn glasses since high school, and three years ago he had to get a stronger prescription. However, since switching to a Paleo lifestyle, he no longer needs to wear his glasses. He has not worn them at all for about three or four months now.")

Of course, as you can tell from her pictures, she also looks great, but let's be realistic for a moment. On her old path of starvation and cardio, looking better was the *whole goal*. If she had somehow managed to achieve her purely aesthetic goal, "she is thin" would have been the only achievement she would have put on her list, and it would have been impossible to maintain.

I had absolutely no influence on the creation of this list. I called Angela and asked her to compile all the benefits she has experienced since I helped her put the final pieces in her puzzle. This was not a chore for her; she is ecstatic about her life now. I can absolutely guarantee you that no amount of fortune or fame would ever be enough to make Angela return to her old unhealthy lifestyle. Has the change been hard? Sometimes. Was it worth it? Hell yes!

I want you to think hard about this. Your happiness may depend on it. Do you want to temporarily turn your body into a flimsy facade that impersonates the true meaning of attractiveness for a mere moment before you return to your frustration? Or do you want to make a list like this of your own? If you answered the way I believe you did, it is imperative that you see the bigger picture. Set your sights on peak health and do not let your focus waver for anything in the world.

# CHAPTER 3
# *temptation's secret plays*

## The Balance Scale

It's time to look at some cold, hard facts. Don't worry—I'll get to the advice in a moment. Everything I teach my clients is quantifiable, and sometimes it stings when we assess the truths. For example, if you have a sugar addiction that is hindering your progress, your desire to appease your cravings outweighs your desire to get healthy and fit. If you do not like meat and it is hindering your progress, flavor is more important to you than results. If you do not like to move your body the way it expects to be moved, your desire to avoid exercise is more important to you than your goals. Nobody can tell you that your stance on these things is wrong or what you should value in your life, but you can either acknowledge your position consciously or live in denial. Facts are facts. When you want Thing A badly enough, you will never let Thing B stand in your way.

Here is a common scenario to help drive this point home. Jane Frustrated-Person meets with me for the first time and is brought to tears when I ask her about her goals. Her frustration clearly runs very deep and she is fed up with her body. When she is taught the ins and outs of Paleo nutrition and proper exercise, Jane becomes excited and marches down this new path, happy and motivated. A couple of months go by and it becomes apparent to me that Jane is not getting the results she should be getting, so I start questioning her to find out why. "What's going on?" I ask her. "You seem to be struggling. Are you eating a solid Paleo diet?" Invariably, the answer is, "I'm trying!"

I can see desperation on Jane's face, but I am forced to push her a little anyway. "*How* are you trying?" I ask.

"I have removed most of the grains from my diet," Jane says. "And I only eat a little bread here and there. Sugar is gone completely—except when I crave ice cream."

Let's analyze this situation, looking at nothing but the facts and removing all emotion. First, eating is an action that requires conscious, purposeful movement on the part of the eater. Usually, at least one hand is required to guide food to the mouth, and then chewing ensues, followed by swallowing. I know of no situation in which these things might happen in this order by accident. Therefore, you cannot *try* to eat. You can eat, or you cannot eat, but there is no trying. *Trying* denotes the possibility of failure. If you say to yourself, "I'm going to eat that grape," there really is no chance of failure unless you choke on the grape and die. You can, however, try to get over a cold, or try to lift a heavy object, or try to pass a test, or even try to lose body fat. But you cannot try to eat or try not to eat. I know it sounds like I am being facetious, but bear with me. To form a workable method of escape from this madness you have to understand when you are oversimplifying the process and not thinking things through. There is no trying when it comes to decisions about what you are going to eat, only varying levels of motivation.

Let me give you another example. Let's pretend that you are a smoker and you are *trying* to quit so you can be a better parent to your kids. Smoking is a serious addiction and quitting is certainly hard, but it is a decision nonetheless and I can prove it. What if I handed you definitive proof that your very next cigarette was guaranteed to give you lung cancer and that you would be dead within a year, leaving your small children to fend for themselves? You would instantly be a nonsmoker. In fact, nobody you have ever held the slightest bit of respect for would ever smoke another cigarette under those circumstances. How is such a remarkable feat possible? Did the biochemical aspects of nicotine addiction magically change with the delivery of this sobering news? Of course not. But your motivation just shot up to unchartable levels.

Here is the same concept from another angle. Have you ever had one of those days when you just could not drag yourself off the couch? Friends may even have called inviting you to join them in activities that would normally launch you out the door, but you could not muster the energy. You were highly motivated to stay on the couch all day. This is truly what you wanted to do, and you were not even willing to *try* to do anything else. Just for fun, let's add a new element to the story and say that your gas stove explodes and your kitchen is suddenly ablaze. Of course you would bolt out of the house like Carl Lewis circa 1984. Did your motivation to stay on the couch change? Not really. It was simply outweighed by your motivation to live. When lying on the couch was your top priority, that is exactly what you did, and you did not have to *try*. When saving your own life was your top priority, that is exactly what you did, and again there was no *trying* involved.

Now back to Jane. When she succumbs to sugar cravings, or any other bad-food temptation, she is making a decision. She has never been held at gunpoint by a suicidal carton of ice cream insistent upon ending its life by forcing her to eat it. On the contrary, she encounters an opportunity to do something she will regret and a choice is made. In her head, the decision might sound like this: "That looks yummy. I am going to eat that." Keeping everything this simple is exactly why change has always been so complicated. We need to go deeper.

If I were to ask Jane to make a list of everything that drove her to pick up her phone and call me before our first meeting, her list would look something like this:

- *I hate the way I look.*
- *Clothes shopping is miserable.*
- *I want to look good for my vacation/wedding/class reunion/graduation/ naked pride parade/etc.*

If I prod her a bit, we could probably extend the list by adding reasons like these:

- *I have no energy.*
- *I can't sleep.*
- *I get out of breath climbing my stairs.*
- *I get migraines.*
- *My stomach always hurts.*
- *Two hours of yard work destroys me for the whole weekend.*
- *I've got pain in my foot/ankle/knee/hip/back/shoulder/head/earlobe/ eyelash/etc.*

That is a decent list of complaints and definitely plenty of reasons to want to change. The next step is to take a look at the list of benefits involved in consuming ice cream. Jane's list would look like this:

- *Ice cream tastes good.*

Hmmm. That list looks a little short in comparison to the first one, but let's keep moving. Jane now has two lists, actually on paper, to fuel her "To Ice Cream or Not To Ice Cream" debate. If we understand that both of Jane's lists are very real to her, each time she caves in and eats ice cream we know that the decision in her head should logically sound like this: "That looks yummy. I want to eat that more than I want to never cry again over the way I look, feel, and perform."

I can comfortably say that I have never encountered anyone in my entire career who would consciously make the decision Jane just made, and Jane would never have consciously made it, either. Yet the decision was made. Why? There are two possibilities, and a combination of the two is most likely.

First, Jane never weighs these choices. She acts on impulse alone. If she were to create an imaginary balance scale in her mind and weigh all the things that make her miserable against all the benefits of ice cream consumption, her scale would crash down on the side of reason, and temporary ice cream insanity would be avoided every time. From there she could make a rational decision about whether cheating is worth it this one time, instead of acting without thinking and regretting it later.

The second major problem for Jane is that she does not *really* believe she can attain her goals. In truth, everything else on her misery list pales when compared with her first item: "I hate the way I look." Her perspective is badly distorted, and she doesn't realize that item number one would vanish if she aimed for health instead. To make matters worse, each of her ill-conceived attempts to look better have ended in failure in the past, further damaging her self-esteem and her ability to visualize anything that resembles success. If she is destined for failure anyway, why deprive herself of foods that give her a moment of happiness? More on this subject later.

Now for the advice. Obviously, these facts, while inarguable, are not so easily rationalized away, and we all have our moments of weakness. However, the imaginary scale is a tool used by those who have successfully reached their goals. They may not actually picture a scale in their minds, but they do weigh the pros and cons before making a decision regarding their nutrition. Asking them, "Why don't you eat cake?" will result in answers like, "I don't want to feel like I got kicked in the gut by a donkey." Or, "I don't want to negate any of my hard work in the gym or my diligence at the dinner table." Or, "I'm full of meat." OK, that last one was more of a physical condition than a rational decision, but the other two make perfect sense.

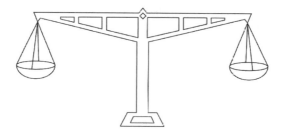

Since I am asking you to create a new habit, I would like you to install an imaginary balance scale in your mind. For those of you who are, like me, not very imaginative, you can use this one.

All that remains is for you to use your newly installed measuring apparatus to weigh the value of your various spontaneous desires against the value of your goals each time you face a precarious decision. The important factor here is taking a moment to consider your options and the consequences. If you still decide in favor of immediate gratification, there should be no self-deprecation afterward. You weighed your options and made a conscious decision. Move on.

The good news is that Paleo nutrition, along with exercise that uses the same logic, will almost always reward you with some modicum of motivating results in just a couple of weeks. Then you will no longer need to have faith alone in the things you place on your scale to weigh against temptation. You will have tangible reasons to stand strong.

Once again, perspective will save the day. When you understand that physical attractiveness is an extension of health, rational decisions win by a landslide because aesthetic goals fill only one small line on a rather extensive list of reasons to stay the course. It's all about health. Hmm, I think I might have said that already.

## Taste and Flavor

I am intrigued by flavor and the human sense of taste. Taste is only one of our five senses, but it wields far more power than any of our other senses.

Humans have evolved five tastes: bitter, sour, salty, sweet, and umami. Each serves a specific purpose and did not evolve by accident. OK, technically everything evolves by accidental mutation, but useful mutations often stick around in the gene pool because of the advantage they offer the organism they evolved in. In the case of the human sense of taste, we are generally drawn to things that sustain us and generally repelled by things that might harm us. Each taste is remarkable and deserves a quick once-over.

Bitterness is the easiest taste for humans to detect, which is great because it often indicates toxicity. Many poisonous plants are bitter, and evolving taste receptors that tell us to spit them out is an asset indeed. At low levels, bitterness is actually palatable and enjoyable. Coffee is a good example of a palatable level of bitterness.

Sour taste indicates acidity and is palatable relative to the acidic dose. Raw lemons approach the limit of desirable sourness for most of us, but fruits like grapefruit are loved by many. Hydrochloric acid, not so much. The more acidic the food (or chemical), the more sour its taste. If something is unbearably sour, it is probably acidic enough to be harmful.

We are drawn to salty flavors because sodium and potassium are necessary electrolytes for human survival. Electrolyte balance is important for cell function, and electrolytes are essential for muscle contraction. The parts of us that must conduct electrical current owe their functionality to electrolytes.

In nature, sweetness tends to mean a source of dense nutrients and digestible calories. Wandering through a jungle tasting things (not recommended!) might result in the consumption of bananas and the rejection of banana leaves. Some amino acids, like alanine and serine, are also sweet, which means meat is also made more desirable by our ability to taste sweetness.

The word "umami" is Japanese and is loosely translated as "good taste." Umami can be described as savory and meaty, and while umami taste is present in some vegetables, it appears to have evolved to make us desire protein. Since consumption of meat is very likely why we evolved our big human brains, umami is definitely a valuable taste.

Now that we have a very basic understanding of our five tastes, it is important to make note of how badly these tastes, and especially sweetness, have been abused in our modern processed foods. Candy and baked goods have very little nutritional value, yet their palatability is very high. In these modern foods, flavors have been extracted from the reasons that we evolved the tastes for them, concentrated, and returned to us to be consumed for pleasure alone. When food becomes a source of pleasure without nutritional value, it's a big problem. Remember, we did not evolve our sense of taste because nature knew that cake would be invented in the future and we needed to be ready. Our five tastes evolved so that we would desire the foods that will keep us alive and healthy.

At the end of the day, taste is simply one sense among five. So why do we let it torment us so? Would you, for example, be willing to sacrifice the way you look, feel, or perform if it meant you could witness more beautiful sunsets? Would you gain thirty pounds so you could listen to more of your favorite music? Would you shorten your life by decades to smell more flowers? "Of course not!" you say. "Now you're just being ridiculous!" Am I? A great many of us have sacrificed our physical well-being, gained weight, and shortened our lives to appease nothing more than our sense of taste. Why are we not willing to pay such a high price to deepen the pleasures our other senses afford?

When you eat chocolate, do you do so because you like the way it feels in your mouth, or the way it slides down your throat, or the way it feels in your stomach? No, you eat chocolate simply because you love the way it tastes. All junk food has the same basic characteristics: very high palatability and very low nutritional value. Go ahead and pick your favorite and make a list of all the reasons you eat it. I will help you get started.

_____ tastes good.

Short but comprehensive. I have to admit, when I first came to the realization that the lion's share of our health problems are a result of our barely conscious need to appease one measly sense with no other reward in sight, I felt a little silly. "How can that be?" I asked myself. But I had no answer. I am certainly quite guilty of this irrational behavior myself. Our sense of taste has been hijacked and turned against us. As the owner of a sentient mind, taste seems unworthy of even a pimple to me, yet many people literally trade their health and ultimately their lives for it.

I realize that the science-minded among you are probably reading this while screaming, "What about dopamine, you dope!" so let's go there for a moment. Dopamine is basically our primary reward hormone. This is an oversimplification, but dopamine evolved in large part to make us repeat behaviors that are rewarding. Drugs like cocaine act upon dopamine and cause all the good feelings of reward without us having to actually do anything to deserve it. We then have a strong desire to repeat the actions that led to the release of dopamine and we become addicted. When we eat food, especially highly palatable food, we experience this same dopamine reward response. This is great if the food that produced the reward response is nutrient-dense and promotes health, but alas, this is not always the case. When we eat garbage foods, they stimulate a reward response via dopamine that makes it highly likely that we will repeat this behavior, except that the behavior being reinforced is actually detrimental to our health instead of beneficial. This amazing system designed to keep us alive and healthy has been dismantled and turned into something that looks very much like drug addiction, except that food addiction is socially acceptable, maybe even socially encouraged.

When we factor in the dopamine reward response, we could say that once we are addicted to processed junk we are not just eating it for flavor anymore; we are also eating it to chase the dopamine response. However, high palatability is necessary to get the whole addiction process started. Think about it—have you ever binged by eating a pound of broccoli? What about steak? No, none of us have. We go straight for processed carbohydrates.

We could dig deep enough into the science behind this stuff to mire ourselves in it, but this book is about changing your perspective. Don't get me wrong, I love biochemistry and physiology as they apply to nutrition and fitness, but others have already written books on those subjects. They do not need to be rehashed on these pages. It is, however, important that we understand when we have been silly. Appeasing one sense to the point of addiction qualifies as such, in my opinion.

I am in no way insinuating that the foods we eat should not be flavorful. Consuming only bland, flavorless foods would probably cause enough depression to shorten our lives anyway. I am merely suggesting that food reward should be justified by nutrient-dense foods that increase vitality, not modern processed crap. Fix the system and get it back to doing what it evolved to do—making us feel good when we eat things that nourish us.

One amazing benefit of Paleo nutrition is that in short order your sense of taste will improve and you will begin to thoroughly enjoy foods that you may currently find uninteresting. This is because there are diminishing returns on the hyperpalatable junk foods you may have become accustomed to, and it takes more and more intense flavors to blow your hair back after a while. Once separated from these foods for a short time, nearly everyone reports experiencing an increase in the flavor of foods that had seemed pedestrian for years. One of my awesome clients, Katie, said, "Carrots suddenly seemed so sweet after sticking to Paleo for a while." You probably just rolled your eyes at that quote, but I double-dog dare you to try it and see what happens.

The take-home message here is that when we distill it all down, we are left with a simple question: Is flavor worth any amount of suffering to you? If you answered yes, that's OK, and nobody can tell you that you are wrong, but please measure and quantify your answer clearly in your head. How much are you willing to suffer just to be able to say "Yum"? If your answer is, "very little," then it is time to break your addiction. If you find it worthwhile to have birthday cake at a party from time to time, I am certainly not going to judge you, but throw it on the balance scale in your mind first. I know your health and fitness goals are important to you, too. They deserve a fair trial.

# Emotional Eating

If you understand the point I just made about flavor, you know that when we eat highly palatable junk food, we get a dopamine response that urges us to repeat this behavior. Therefore, it is quite possible to become addicted to junk food. This means we technically have another reason to eat poorly besides flavor alone. Still, I am sticking to my flavor argument because I am asking you to use your sentient mind to think about what is really going on when you are drawn to eat that way, and it all starts with flavor.

The fact that dopamine is a feel-good hormone makes emotional eating extremely common. The essence of emotional eating is often escape. If you are an alcoholic who has trudged through a tough day, you turn to alcohol for escape. If food is the avenue by which you appease your dopamine cravings, you will binge when life gets you down.

A client once told me that when she was depressed she would "suddenly" find herself sitting on her couch surrounded by empty junk food bags and boxes. Naturally more depression followed all the self-abuse she then inflicted on herself: "Why did you eat all that crap? You're disgusting!" Bouts like these are not easy to recover from, especially when you can't ask yourself to leave.

Sometimes emotional eating is about happy memories and trying to re-capture moments in our past that we hold dear. If your warm childhood memories tend to include food like fried chicken and Mom's homemade apple pie, sometimes all you want is to eat those foods in the hope of re-experiencing how happy and carefree life was in those days. I am totally sympathetic to the reality that food is capable of tugging at your heartstrings. I just want you to understand what is really going on so you can circumvent these subconscious tugs and achieve the level of health and fitness you desire.

The pursuit of the next dopamine-induced happy spell may be keeping you from reaching your goals. I would not be surprised if a drug was eventually designed to block dopamine when we eat so that we would lose our food reward response and no longer want to binge. In fact, a drug like this may already exist, but I am not sure and I don't really care. I predict that the problem would be getting people to take it. People usually do not understand all the forces at work; they eat junk, they feel good for the short while it takes to hit their stomachs, and to hell with the details. Blocking dopamine would have the same effect as not eating junk food. It makes a lot more sense to find another way to feel good.

The answer is accomplishment. I will venture to say that you have probably never experienced a time when you were simultaneously proud of yourself and depressed. I could be wrong, but I can personally say that it is true for me. When I accomplish something, especially something important to me or something pertaining to a current goal, I feel like a million bucks. Therefore, I think I can safely say that doing something good for yourself just might be rewarding enough to replace the false reward you are looking for when you eat junk food.

As with our mental balance scale, I am again asking you to take a moment to think instead of acting on impulse. When you find yourself feeling low and circling like a hawk preparing to swoop down and snatch an unsuspecting cream-filled doughnut or ten, remind yourself of what is really going on and find a way to do something that will actually bring about happy results and not merely a cheap imitation of them.

Now for some really good news. If you are serious about your goals and truly want to improve your health and fitness with all your heart, simply resisting temptation is the answer to your dreams. I cannot count the times I have heard a client excitedly exclaim, "I went to a friend's house for a party last weekend and there was junk food everywhere, but I didn't have a single bite!" These self-satisfied boasts are always accompanied by big smiles and lots of pride. And why should this person not be happy? He faced tough odds and made the right decision. I say, "Hell yeah!" and commence with high-five-ory!

When I walked you through that scenario just now, did you feel a little bit of the excitement you felt after a big accomplishment in the past? I got a little amped up just writing about it! Did you ever feel that good after you killed a bag of Oreos? No, of course not. The immediate gratification we get when our emotions drive us to eat junk food can be better described as temporary relief from whatever was bothering us, but it does not take us all the way to happy. I think happy is better.

# CHAPTER 4

# the wrong way to keep score

## Scale Addiction

Here is a nice little piece of craziness: In a species that judges physical attractiveness visually, the bathroom scale has become the unequivocal, unparalleled tool for measuring aesthetics. Which is to say that measuring gravity's effect on your body and then assuming this measurement to be relevant to your physical attractiveness is the norm. The astute reader will notice that there is not one single place in this book where I mention how much weight someone lost. Why? Because weight is misleading and irrelevant.

Chances are good that you picked up this book because you want to change the way you look. I understand completely, but I am doing my best to convince you that the path to looking great is all about improving your health. I am not disagreeing with your desire to look better, just pointing out that you have probably been going about it all wrong.

On this subject, however, I am totally calling you out. Weighing yourself to measure your progress is ridiculous. Allow me to explain, first with some logical silliness, then with inarguable proof.

Some points to ponder for those of you who love your scale and think there is such a thing as an "ideal weight":

I am fairly sure that I weigh about 175 pounds as I write this; I am not positive because *I do not weigh myself*. If I were to travel to Mars, I would weigh approximately 64 pounds. Would I be more attractive there? On Jupiter I would weigh 401 pounds. Would I be less attractive there than here on Earth?

Have you ever been on a blind date? Did you weigh that person when you first met? No? Then how did you know if he or she was attractive?

When I was a teenager trolling the mall in suburban America, we did not carry scales to weigh the young girls we drooled over. We were capable of acting like complete idiots without the need of such tools.

Once upon a time, a new female client who is 5 feet 5 inches tall, told me that she believed her ideal weight was 115 pounds. I asked her if she wanted to qualify this concept with more information and she said no. So I clarified for her that she was essentially saying that 5 foot 5 inches and 115 pounds is a formula for attractiveness. Of course that is complete nonsense. There are, without question, many women with those numbers who absolutely do not have great looking bodies. It seems even more absurd if you apply the same logic to men. Would anyone ever assume that all men look great at 5 foot 11 inches and 180 pounds? No way! Those numbers could apply to every physique from well-muscled to chicken legs and a potbelly.

Most of us have been in love at some point. Remember the beginning? Think back to when you were both so infatuated with each other that you floated around with your heads in the clouds. Did your love interest ever weigh you or ask you how much you weighed? So you mean to tell me that you weighed yourself every day, always knowing your exact weight to the ounce, and yet this person was somehow able to judge your physical appearance without ever knowing that number? Impossible!

According to scale-addiction logic, men all over the world are frustrated with *Playboy* magazine to the point of screaming. *Playboy* gives all the relevant measurements of their centerfolds except weight. I picture angry men gathered on the sidewalk outside the Playboy mansion yelling, "Damn you, Hugh Hefner! How can I tell if this woman is beautiful if you will not tell me what she weighs!"

All right, I'm done being ludicrous, but you have to admit, all of those points are valid. If we want to get nitpicky about the semantics, we'd say that people aren't trying to lose *weight*; they are trying to lose *fat*. This is worth noting, but I didn't bring up this subject to argue semantics. There are much more important factors at stake here, the most important of which is the fact that the vast majority of people in the Western world are measuring their attractiveness, success, failure, and happiness using a tool that is guaranteed to betray them at some point in their journey to becoming fit and healthy. I understand that right now your inner voice is stammering, "But ... but ... but ...," because you are addicted to your scale and the valid information you have convinced yourself it has to offer. I hope you don't think I would come to this discussion unprepared. Sit down and hold on tight.

I spent a good chunk of my career waiting patiently for the picture on the next page to come into my life, so desperately did I long to put this scale fallacy to bed. I submit for your approval, exhibit A: Deb at a size 12 on the left and at a size 6 on the right.

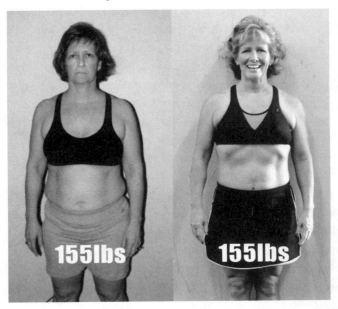

Yes, you read that right. Deb weighed 155 pounds in both pictures. Be sure to scrutinize every little detail in those pictures, comparing every feature of each one to the other. When you are done and your inner voice stops telling you that I am lying to you, we will move on.

In the fitness industry we tend to hear "Muscle weighs more than fat!" repeated ad nauseam, but when evidence like these pictures is produced, the response is always something like, "Wow! That's amazing! Muscle weighs more than fat! Who knew?" I find it interesting that such a well-accepted truth has been so thoroughly ignored that even the majority of those in the fitness industry chanting "Muscle weighs more than fat!" think the scale is the essential means of measuring attractiveness.

You may not yet be convinced, so let's stay with this concept. What if Deb came to me weighing 200 pounds and told me she wanted to get down to 155? Which body pictured above do you think she would prefer? Do you think she would have been satisfied with the one on the left? Look at her face. She is ecstatic with her body on the right, while on the left she can barely stand to have her picture taken. But according to scale-addict logic, she would have reached her goal with the body in either picture and I could happily chalk her up as another job well done.

Here's the lesson: Goals based on weight are too vague to be useful. If I had given you only her measurements (waist, hips, thighs, bust, etc.) with no weight and no photos, there is absolutely no doubt in my mind which 155-pound Deb you would have chosen as the more aesthetically appealing. Yet, if you looked in the mirror and saw a body like Deb's on the left, you'd probably say, "Damn, I need to lose some weight!" From there, the process would involve weighing yourself regularly to see if you were making progress. Now you have undeniable evidence that defies such reasoning. *You do not want to lose weight!* Pursuing a number on your scale is *not* the path to success—it is the path to frustration. I'll go out on a limb here, but I'm guessing that frustration is not your goal.

I will concede that the number on the scale will go down if you have a lot of weight to lose. The problem is that the scale will not tell you when it is no longer serving your goal, and in reality it is never entirely accurate. Nobody loses all her fat before she begins gaining muscle, and Paleo with proper exercise will always result is some muscle gain in sedentary individuals. This means that the scale is hiding some of your results right from the start. For example, a loss of fifteen pounds of fat accompanied by a gain of five pounds of muscle will look like only a ten-pound loss according to the scale. Eventually, when enough fat is lost, the number on the scale will stop going down, and maybe even start going up, while pant sizes will still be decreasing. At this point it would be nice if the scale said, "OK, I'm useless now. Go do something else." Alas, we are not so lucky. Without being given fair warning, what would you do in this situation if you had not reached your *ideal weight*?

In a past life I worked for a fitness company that required all of its trainers to keep meticulous records of every client's weight. On two separate occasions clients arrived bubbly and ecstatic because their pants were nearly falling off from all the fat they had lost, only to be driven to tears after stepping on the scale. Both times I wanted to scream. It was maddening to watch these people beat themselves up after making such great progress. Their scale addiction ran so deep that a stupid number was all that mattered to them. You might think that these examples are a bit extreme, and maybe you would be happy with size lost despite weight gained, but I would bet a stack of cash that there is a scale in your bathroom at this very moment. Do you cross a lot of rickety bridges with very specific weight limits? If not, then what do you use your scale for?

Now for some much more rational advice. I think it's safe to say that we have established that nobody is technically trying to lose weight but is, rather, trying to lose fat. We have also established that we all judge physical attraction visually. Our eyes can see the size of a body, but they cannot measure weight. Therefore, the only tools that make any sense to use are the measuring tape and the mirror. If you have fat-loss goals and the circumference of your waist, hips, thighs, etc. decreases, or your clothing sizes go down, you have made progress, regardless of what the scale may try to interject. Even better, if you look in the mirror and like what you see better than what you saw when you started your new regime, do not let the scale have an opinion on the matter.

I cannot close this subject without sharing what I consider the best possible scenario. In my dream world, all the concepts in this book are understood by everyone and people don't measure anything about their bodies except physical capacity. Everyone focuses on a Paleo lifestyle, celebrating every good decision in his diet and every new accomplishment in his fitness, and everyone gets hot by accident as he pursues peak health. When aesthetics are improved, they are simply added to a long list of benefits describing a fantastic new lease on life.

I know these are unrealistic expectations. Most of us love to quantify things. But at least promise me that you will ditch the scale in favor of the more useful data provided by the measuring tape and the mirror. Maybe you will find it easier to stay the course and bring your own list of benefits to fruition. An inanimate object that spends its life lying on the bathroom floor next to your toilet should not be given the power to break your heart.

## BMI? Seriously?

The gold standard for determining healthy body weight as far as modern medicine is concerned is the body mass index (BMI). Your BMI is calculated by dividing your weight by the square of your height. In other words, Deb's BMI is exactly the same in both of the pictures on page 60. BMI also teaches us that every professional male bodybuilder is morbidly obese, and probably so are most female bodybuilders, at least at their off-season weight. If you are sincerely attempting to get healthy and fit, please do not take BMI seriously. In fact, you might want to consider ignoring anyone who takes BMI seriously. Seriously.

# CHAPTER 5
# don't change the rules

## The System Is Broken

Dallas and Melissa Hartwig wrote the amazing and popular Paleo-nutrition guide *It Starts with Food*. That title really resonated with me because I have yet to discover a situation regarding health and fitness in which this is not true.

Everything about health and fitness is about inputs. Nutrition, sleep, exercise, and stress are the biggies, but I must say that I agree with the Hartwigs: Food is at the top of the list. Interestingly, "common knowledge" gives none of these things due credit for their effects on health. If we resign ourselves to the mainstream perspective, we might come to believe that noninfectious diseases and disorders are simply in the cards we're dealt and that there is nothing we can do to avoid them. This perspective is a huge problem for us but a huge benefit for those who would profit from our ill health.

As I write this, the United States is consuming more pharmaceutical drugs than any other country by a wide margin, yet the CIA World Factbook ranks us fiftieth for life expectancy at birth. So, I have a silly question: *What the hell are all those drugs for?* We are sucking down pharmaceuticals at an alarming rate, but nearly all the other first world countries have higher life expectancies than we do. If this doesn't make you mad, you are not paying attention.

Actually, it is not very difficult to see how we got here. Prevention is not profitable, and researching how to prevent disease is a great way to make sure there is never any return on research dollars. If people understood how to prevent themselves from getting sick, there wouldn't be as much need for drugs—that is, for pharmaceutical companies to make big bucks. Thus, we don't hear much advice about how to keep ourselves from getting, say, cancer, heart disease, and type 2 diabetes, but we hear all about the drugs designed to *treat* them.

As a hypothetical example, let's pretend that the world's richest man financed a study definitively proving that vanilla ice cream is the sole cause of cancer in humans. Let's also pretend that this study cost him $300 million, which is a reasonable estimation. How can he see a return on his investment? Can he attach meters to our mouths and charge us every time we don't eat vanilla ice cream? Probably not. Everyone would quit eating vanilla ice cream and quit getting cancer without ever purchasing a single thing from him, and his $300 million would be gone forever. Big Pharma finances the majority of research, and Big Pharma is an *industry* composed of *corporations* that are obligated to their shareholders to maximize *profits*. There are no conspiracies at work here, just simple economics. The problems arise when people buy into the marketing hype and begin to believe that these companies employ only angels whose sole purpose on earth is to keep us all happy and healthy until we each reach our one-hundredth birthday. In reality they put on their pants and go to work each morning to make money just like you.

## Put the Knife Down!

Here's a news flash for you: Treatment is for sick people. You don't want treatment. You don't want to get sick. Here's another news flash for you: You have control over your own health. Genetic predispositions that guarantee death by any particular noninfectious disease are very rare. Let's put that another way: We do not get sick by accident; we choose the inputs that determine the level of health and vitality we experience in our lives. Don't kid yourself: You are not a victim; you just aren't asking the right questions, and mainstream medicine isn't asking them, either.

Let me give you an example of how the current mainstream thinking is so badly warped. John Typical-Patient goes to see his doctor because he has terrible heartburn and it is keeping him awake at night. He tells his doc about his suffering and before he can finish his story he is handed a prescription for Prilosec, a drug that is actually quite effective at relieving heartburn that comes from acid reflux. Therefore, we can infer from his doctor's response that John Typical-Patient's Prilosec gland was on the blink and that his body was not manufacturing enough of this particular drug. At this point you are probably thinking, "Don't be ridiculous—of course that is not what his doctor meant!" But if you think about it, there is not really any other way to look at the situation. Heartburn is a symptom, not a disease, and even

GERD (gastroesophageal reflux disease) does not happen by accident. The same can be said for headaches, dizziness, insomnia, muscle pain, diarrhea, constipation, lack of appetite, memory loss, skin rashes, itchy eyes, coughing, sneezing, vomiting, and virtually every other symptom that might send you to your doctor.

Make no mistake: I am by no means trying to vilify all doctors or say that you shouldn't check in with your doctor if you exhibit any of the aforementioned symptoms. But I am saying that treating symptoms is a lot like whittling on your finger while looking for a better bandage. What you really need is to put the damn knife down!

So, business as usual in modern medicine looks like this: Some sort of input causes a problem, this problem results in at least one symptom, the symptom is treated with man-made inputs (drugs), which invariably come with side effects, and the source of the problem is usually not addressed at all. How can this possibly make sense?

Look, I am not preaching a hippie "Don't put chemicals in your body" position here, even though that is good advice. What I am saying, pleading really, is that treating symptoms downstream of the real problem is madness and should never have gotten this far. For a look at just how counterproductive this can be, allow me to give you yet another example. If you suffer from headaches on a regular basis, you might take ibuprofen for some relief, and it might actually work. Since it has never occurred to you that your headaches could be a *symptom* of something more serious, you keep on trucking without giving the matter a second thought. You get headaches, ibuprofen fixes them, end of story. Unfortunately, the cause of your headaches keeps on trucking too. What if the cause is high blood pressure from borderline type 2 diabetes? This could be easily managed with proper diet and exercise, but you essentially allow it to fester because your symptom is under control. Now you are at increased risk of a heart attack, among other things. To make matters worse, the ibuprofen comes with side effects, like gastrointestinal damage and … increased risk of myocardial infarction, known on the mean streets by the alias Heart Attack. Doesn't it make a lot more sense to figure out what is actually causing your headaches so you can avoid this whole mess?

Maybe none of these examples apply to you, but I hope you are beginning to get my point. When we understand that an external stimulus is almost always required to reach a state of ill health, then we can also understand that the external stimulus is the first thing that must be addressed. Just as in my finger-whittling example, if you are repeatedly hitting yourself in the head with a hammer, aspirin might help, but I bet you can come up with a better solution.

As usual, the right perspective holds all the answers. The next time something goes wrong with your body, ask "What caused that?" until you are positive there are no more answers.

What's wrong? Headaches. What caused that? High blood pressure. What caused that? Borderline type 2 diabetes. What caused that? Standard American Diet. Hurray! Now we have something we can work with!

"Hold on a minute!" you say. "I don't have the knowledge or the resources to answer those questions on my own, and my doc just wants to give me drugs!" This may be true, but your hands are not tied. While virtually everything you could ever want to know about physiology, biochemistry, and every known disease is available somewhere out there on the Interwebs, most people do not have the time or energy to devote to the self-education required to find their own answers. If this is you, you still have one amazing answer available to you: Start with Paleo nutrition!

Regardless of your symptoms or disease, it always makes sense to begin by giving your body human food and eliminating all the processed garbage. Chances are very good that the garbage is what caused the problem in the first place, but the good news is that you do not have to know for sure. Whenever anyone makes a serious play for strict Paleo, invariably problems at least improve, if they're not completely resolved. The only question is, *Why would you not try?*

Throughout my career I have encountered people suffering terribly from various ailments while eating a horrible, deleterious diet and patiently waiting for the next drug that will finally rescue them from their anguish. If I have been doing my job here, you have begun to see the error in this way of thinking.

Sometimes things get broken and drugs will still be necessary, but at least you will not be treating symptoms if you have asked "What caused that?" enough times. In many cases, a change in nutrition and lifestyle can make an enormous difference, even with some of the havoc-wreaking heavy-hitter diseases.

# *Erika*

When Erika was almost sixteen, she woke up one morning to find that the pinky finger on her left hand was numb. The next morning her pinky and ring fingers were numb. Each consecutive morning added more numbness until her entire arm and the left side of her torso were numb in about a week. Initially, her mother thought that maybe she had a pinched nerve, either from carrying her heavy school bag or possibly from playing sports. Erika said, "It got to a point where I couldn't even raise my arm anymore and if someone poked me in the arm at school I wouldn't even notice because I couldn't feel it."

Erika's mother decided to take her to an urgent-care facility. The first thing the doctor asked was whether Erika had taken any illicit drugs. The question makes perfect sense, but innocent, young Erika was shocked. After a thorough examination, the doctor was stumped and referred her to a local hospital, where she ended up spending the next two weeks. After lots of testing, the doctors concluded that she had either multiple sclerosis (MS) or acute disseminated enchephalomyelitis (ADEM). Erika and her doctors were hoping for ADEM because it is temporary, with full recovery in as many as 75 percent of all cases, whereas multiple sclerosis has no cure and could mean total debilitation over time. She was sent home with prescriptions for Neurontin for neuropathic pain and Prednisone for inflammation.

Erika had some notable side effects from these drugs. "Because of the Prednisone, I gained ten pounds in my midsection in about a month," she said. "I have permanent stretch marks from that. And I had never had acne before, but now it was everywhere. The Neurontin was supposed to help with my numbness, but it never worked, and I actually had some hallucinations from it. It also caused severe joint pain—like wake-up-in-the-middle-of-the-night-crying kind of joint pain—and the doctor eventually said I could quit taking it."

Months passed with no improvement, lots of MRIs, and still no official diagnosis. Finally, before yet another MRI, one of her doctors told her that if her situation appeared to be getting worse, she had MS, and if it stayed the same or improved it was ADEM. "I was called in earlier than my next appointment, so I knew something was wrong," Erika said. "On December 8, 2008, I was diagnosed with multiple sclerosis."

At this point, Erika was prescribed Avonex, an interferon drug, with the hope of slowing the progression of her MS. "I was sixteen years old giving myself an intramuscular injection every week," she said. They hurt a lot!" Interferon drugs also cause flu-like symptoms. Erika would try to administer her shots at night in the hope of sleeping through the nausea, but she did not always get so lucky.

After about a year on Avonex, she was prescribed Rebif instead. Rebif is also an interferon drug, but the shots are subcutaneous (under the skin) instead of intramuscular (in the muscle), and Erika had to give herself injections three times a week rather than once. "The Rebif hurt so much worse than the Avonex, and they seemed to fester under my skin, leaving purple bruises the size of fifty-cent pieces all over my arms and legs," Erika said, gesturing to her entire thigh. "I was so upset that I had to be on this medicine because it was just before summer and I was about to turn eighteen. I didn't want nasty bruises all over my legs, and they didn't go away for weeks."

These drugs can damage the liver as well. "Every three months I would have a liver-function test, which usually isn't necessary unless you are on a scary drug or you are a severe alcoholic." This is a tough reality for an eighteen-year-old kid. The message was crystal clear—*we are treating your disease, but you are paying for it.*

Despite all the drugs, and all the side effects, Erika's MS was getting worse. Her doctors suggested a drug called Tysabri (Natalizumab), which is administered intravenously once a month. The side effects include risk of progressive multifocal leukoencephalopathy (PML), a rare but often fatal disease of the brain. Erika decided the risk was too great and declined to be treated with Tysabri.

In October 2010, I spoke about Paleo nutrition in a class Erika was taking at one of our local colleges. Erika's curiosity was piqued. She decided to try Paleo and began doing some of her own research. The results came quickly. She stopped taking her medications, and in no time her symptoms disappeared.

"On all the medications I still had some numbness," Erika said. "And then after stopping the medications and going Paleo I started to feel better than I had since before my diagnosis."

What comes next infuriates me, so before I go on I would like to say that my intention is not to disrespect the medical community. There are many excellent medical professionals out there. In fact, the Paleo Physicians network (www.paleophysiciansnetwork.com) is a fantastic and ever-growing resource full of them. This is not an attack on all doctors, and I am certainly not suggesting that you should never again seek professional medical help. But please understand that business as usual in mainstream medicine is not OK. That's all I'm saying. OK, back to our story.

Erika currently has no clinical symptoms and the way she feels has dramatically improved, yet ever since she found Paleo, her doctors have told her that her refusal to take drugs means that she has decided to do nothing. In their eyes, she is only crossing her fingers and hoping everything works out. She has explained to them that she changed the way she eats and exercises, but it makes no difference to them. She has stopped taking her prescription medications, which means that her progress is clearly a result of her nutrition and lifestyle changes, but they will not hear of it. One doctor even asked, "So you are just going to do nothing and hope for the best?" Erika told me, "I am absolutely not just hoping for the best. I am taking matters into my own hands by changing my diet and exercise." In this doctor's opinion, not taking a drug is exactly the same as doing nothing, even though doing nothing is exactly what the drugs he had been prescribing had been doing.

Technically, Erika is doing a lot more work by taking responsibility for her own health. It cost her only a few minutes a week to take her drugs as she was instructed. Now she is actively fighting her MS at every meal and every workout. It seems to me that "Do nothing and hope for the best" is a much better description of the medicated route than the route Erika has chosen. Taking a few drugs and continuing to live as usual sounds a lot more like "hoping for the best" than the lifestyle overhaul Erika has undertaken.

I asked Erika if she thinks she has any symptoms that set her apart from me and the rest of the healthy people in the world. She responded, "None at all. But my doctors have a terrible time believing me. They do all these neurological tests on me, as well as test my strength. I always surprise them, but they still don't believe me."

By nature, MS is a disease that impedes the brain's ability to communicate with the body, thereby causing a gradual loss of motor ability. This means that over time Erika should be losing her strength and her ability to use her muscles. Let's see if this is Erika's reality, shall we?

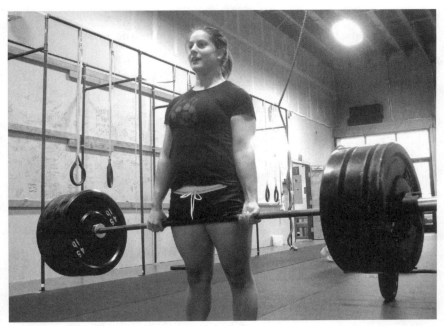

*Erika deadlifting 275-pounds*

Here are Erika's current strength numbers:

Dead Lift: 285 lbs.
Back Squat: 220 lbs.
Shoulder Press: 95 lbs.
Bench Press: 115 lbs.

One of the questions Erika is always asked by her doctors is, "Are you experiencing any weakness?" Ha!

Erika's story warms my heart, and I hope it is helpful to those with multiple sclerosis, but there is a lesson here for everyone. Most people think of MS as a terrifying, life-ending disease because mainstream medicine does not tend to produce results like these. Erika asked "What caused that?" until she couldn't find any more answers, and then she used Paleo and proper exercise to become as healthy as she possibly could. If she had accepted the notion that she got sick by random chance and without the influence of any external inputs, she would still be taking drugs with awful side effects and keeping her fingers crossed. Instead, she began eating in a way that her body understood and gave her brain what it needed to get healthy again.

The example Erika has set for us is powerful because she is such a strong, young woman, and MS is no joke, but her perspective can be adopted by anyone. Please allow me to reiterate—I am not suggesting that we all abandon modern medicine and treat ourselves at home with Paleo. However, I am absolutely suggesting that we avidly hunt for the cause of anything that may ever cause us pain and suffering. I am also suggesting that treatment of noninfectious disease without controlling the inputs makes sense only if you believe that we contract these diseases by pure chance.

Are you with me now? If you take only one thing from this whole book, make it this: You must look upstream from your problems until you know you have reached the source. That rule applies to everything from major diseases to excess fat. In the meantime, start with solid human nutrition, also called the Paleo diet. If research is not your thing, just start with Paleo because you have nothing to lose and everything to gain, and then search for a Paleo-friendly doctor who is willing to help you find the cause of your problems.

## Those Damn Guidelines

In their defense, doctors have specific guidelines that they must follow or risk being sued for malpractice. For example, doctors who are aware that high cholesterol is not the cause of heart disease are on shaky ground when they do what they know is right by not prescribing statin drugs. If a patient who has been told how to eat properly instead of being given a statin still dies of a heart attack, no amount of scientific data on earth will save that doctor's butt in court; following guidelines is what is most important, even when the guidelines have a terrible track record.

While I've been standing atop my soapbox, preaching the merits of searching for the causes of whatever may ail us, this guidelines thing has often been brought up for discussion. I freely admit that following prescribed rules is a valid excuse for doctors and that it often ties their hands, as well as the hands of patients with insurance that limits them to specific doctors within a group known for strict protocols. But red tape is not reason enough to give up and settle for being sick. If you are not getting the help you had hoped for from the medical profession and it is not possible to find more help, you still have one option: It's time to start learning.

We live in a remarkable age. Information moves at mind-boggling speeds, and nearly every piece of data ever discovered is available to everyone with the desire to look for it. Sometimes accurate information can be elusive among the in-your-face misinformation dubbed "common knowledge," but in my experience eventually the truth will come out. You cannot afford to be shuffled off to the Land of Normal by inept guidelines disseminated by a profit-driven medical industry.

## *Will Paleo Help?*

I could never count how many times I have been asked, "Will Paleo help with my [*insert disease or disorder here*]?" The answer is almost always a resounding yes! Will Paleo cure your disease or disorder? I have no idea. Will Paleo have a direct positive effect on your disease or disorder? Again, I can't say for sure. But I can absolutely say that eating foods that your body understands and expects will certainly improve your health, and a healthier body always stands a better chance than an unhealthy one of overcoming obstacles.

As you have already seen through multiple examples in this book, Paleo nutrition has helped many people with many things, in some cases even causing some issues to vanish entirely. These are all anecdotal cases, and I have no idea what will happen to you exactly, but I can promise that you will get healthier. The good news is that if you're wondering whether Paleo will help, and you are seeking relief from a particular disease or disorder, you probably have a higher level of motivation than those who just want a smaller pant size. Here's my advice: Go Paleo and let's see what happens.

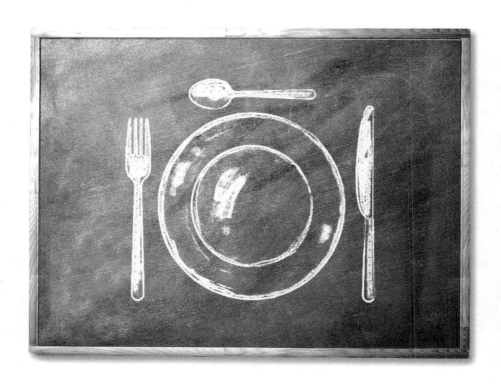

EAT

# CHAPTER 6
## the playing field

### Let's Do It!

Up to this point my sole purpose has been to help you get your head right. I have never seen someone with the right perspective and ample motivation fall short of his goals once he had a good map to success. Here comes the map. I promise not to bury you in science, but we are going all the way back to the beginning. Let's go.

### What Are You?

You and I are humans. More specifically, we are *Homo sapiens*. As such, we can be described as animals, vertebrates, mammals, primates, and hominids. For ease of discussion, let's reduce our taxonomy and simply say that we are animals. I remind you of this because it is a fact that is easily forgotten, and the negative implications of our identity crisis have been extensive.

There are a few basic rules that apply to all animals that are worth discussing early in our journey so that we can understand why some of our expectations about our health may not be as logical as we may think. All animals have the same three goals: to eat, procreate, and try not to die. These things are nonnegotiable, but humans, with our complex minds, have tweaked the details in ways that no other creature has yet considered.

Koalas are herbivores and have been eating eucalyptus leaves for as long as there have been koalas. Wolves are carnivores and have been eating other animals for as long as there have been wolves. These facts are easy to understand, at least until we start talking about humans, and then everyone gets confused for some reason.

No other animal can alter its environment to an extent even remotely approaching that of humans. It is also a fact that we have paid dearly for the changes we have wrought on our environment, and the cost has been to our health. Nearly everything we do in our day-to-day lives is outside the realm of what our bodies expect—from the way we move; to the way we eat; to the way we sleep, sit, play, and work. The selective pressures that molded us armed us with the tools we needed to be strong and capable in a world that quite literally vanished in the last blink of our history. In other words, our modern world is at odds with our primitive bodies. Should we throw up our hands and resign ourselves to sickness, obesity, weakness, and lack of energy? Absolutely not! Thankfully, we can have the best of both of our colliding worlds.

## *Paleo?*

Merriam-Webster defines the word "diet" as follows:

*a.* food and drink regularly provided or consumed
*b.* habitual nourishment
*c.* the kind and amount of food prescribed for a person or animal for a special reason
*d.* a regimen of eating and drinking sparingly so as to reduce one's weight <going on a *diet*>

I do not often use the words "Paleo" and "diet" together because they tend to make people think that I am referring to a diet in the sense of *d* above. Unfortunately, this definition is so prevalent that even many researchers use the word "diet" to mean caloric restriction unless otherwise specified. Wikipedia says that "diet" is "the sum of the food consumed by an organism or group." I like this definition much better, but it still leaves me wanting. In reality, Paleo nutrition simply asks one very important question: What is the natural diet for *Homo sapiens*?

To understand why this question is so important we must start by discussing some basic truths about health and nutrition. First and foremost, it is important to understand that we should really not be using the word "diet" as a verb or an activity. No other creature can be described as "doing a diet" or "dieting." Animals *have* diets. Only humans *do* diets. In light of this fact, I would like to pose my own, additional definition of the word "diet," which Merriam-Webster is free to include as category *e* above:

*A conscious and deliberate change in nutritional intake for the express purpose of reaching a specific goal or goals*

This definition implies a departure from one way of eating in favor of another, which in turn implies that the original way of eating was either flawed or perceived as such. This is why animals in the wild are never seen weighing their portions or omitting specific foods they would otherwise consume. There is no need. The natural diet of the bison, for example, will not cause obesity or disease in bison. It is the same for tigers, hummingbirds, cuttlefish, and crickets. Nature just does not work any other way. Natural selective pressures push every species toward either better means of survival or extinction. Therefore, all creatures eat according to the plan that best promotes their reproductive fitness, and thus the survival of their species. All creatures except humans, that is.

As humans, we have these pesky sentient minds and the ability to intervene on the natural plan. There was a time when we played by the same rules as all the animals. In fact, our diet was molded by nature and natural selection for more than two million years. It was only roughly 10,000 years ago, with the discovery of agriculture, that we decided that we knew better than nature. Technically, we probably were trying to advance our species when we began manipulating nature to grow our own food because it was agriculture that allowed us to settle down in one location and form societies, which eventually led to our escape from many of the selective pressures we faced throughout the rest of our history. Most of us have never even known someone who knows someone who died from falling prey to an animal predator, and we have agriculture, and thereby the overhaul of our environment, to thank for that. Wild lions are indeed a rare sight in cities, even cities in Africa. But natural selection is a powerful force, and there are consequences when you defy the force, consequences in terms of our health and vitality.

When we examine the anthropological record, as well as the indigenous hunter-gatherer tribes living today, we do not find a rate of noninfectious disease that is remotely comparable to modern western societies. Obesity, heart disease, stroke, cancer, type 2 diabetes, rheumatoid arthritis, Alzheimer's, Parkinson's, autism, celiac, Hashimoto's, lupus, cataracts; the list is mountainous and none of these things is found in numbers worth mentioning in people eating a traditional hunter gatherer diet, or anywhere in the animal kingdom for that matter. Once we begin to understand this concept, we are but one small step from understanding the importance of our evolutionary heritage and why ridiculous concepts like severe caloric restriction and the vilification of certain macronutrients have no place in a healthy human diet.

The bottom line is that we had it right when we ate and moved the way natural selective pressures molded us to eat and move. The last time we were all on the same page, without a single human on earth changing the rules, was in the late Paleolithic period, ending approximately 10,000 years ago with the agricultural revolution. Paleo is humans looking back in order to move forward. Paleo is how we can recapture the health and vitality that is our birthright.

## But 'Cavemen' Lived Only Thirty Years!

One of the most common arguments against Paleo nutrition is actually nothing more than a simple misunderstanding. It goes like this: *Why would we want to emulate cavemen when they lived to be only thirty years old?* This sounds like a valid concern, right? While it is true that average life expectancy in the Upper Paleolithic was only a few years past thirty, the keyword here is "average." First of all, without sanitation, hygiene, trauma care, and treatment of infection, life was considerably more perilous. When we throw in high infant-mortality rates and predators, the situation gets especially dire for the wee ones. It is possible that as many as 50 percent of all individuals may not have lived past adolescence, thus the *average* is dragged down. If Paleolithic men and women survived past those sketchy years, they stood a good chance of living well into middle age. Therefore, a life expectancy of about thirty years does not mean that all of our Paleolithic ancestors dropped dead at age thirty.

Once we understand that Paleolithic life expectancy is an average that is heavily affected by a high death rate in early life, using life expectancy as an argument against eating and moving the way we did in the Upper Paleolithic becomes invalid. I doubt that anyone is claiming that food choices and movement patterns were the cause of the high death rate in babies and youth. If dietary choices were killing off the kids, those same choices would have probably killed off the adults, as well.

We are emulating cavemen (I hate that word) because we want to have our cake and eat it, too. We want their health while simultaneously living in a cleaner, safer world, where treatment for would-be life-threatening trauma is almost always nearby. Today, a nasty cut on your hand can be easily cleaned and stitched instead of becoming infected and festering until it ends your life. Our ancient ancestors were not always the pointy tip of the food chain, and they also lived lives in which an accident could easily become a death sentence. Most of us, on the other hand, will not die from any kind of accident. The good news is that the top causes of death in humans today are avoidable. Of course, "avoidable" implies action. If you are willing to make some changes, you can have the health of our ancestors with the comforts our modern world.

## Haven't We Evolved to Eat These Modern Foods?

A common question the Paleo-proficient hear when telling someone about Paleo for the first time goes something like this: If we have been eating these modern foods for 10,000 years, haven't we evolved to eat them? Again, this question is just a simple misunderstanding, this time of natural selection.

In reality, we will probably never fully adapt to our modern diet because the diseases it promotes do not tend to kill us until well after the years of reproductive fitness. Therefore, if genetics that allow for consequence-free consumption were present in any individual, those genes would not give that individual a reproductive advantage. Let me translate: You could eat nothing but fast food and still have a dozen kids. Nature does not care if you live until your ninetieth birthday or your fortieth birthday, as long as you make babies. To help you understand this concept, let's look at the rapid evolution that occurred in some genetic lines in relation to lactose tolerance.

Technically speaking, we all have the genes for lactose tolerance because we begin our lives with the need to digest the lactose in our mother's milk. However, as we progress out of infancy this gene is sometimes "turned off" and our lactose tolerance can be lost. It is likely that this maturity-related change happened in almost all humans prior to the domestication of the animals that provide us with milk.

Picture a situation in which agrarian people (sustaining themselves through agriculture) have settled in one place, possibly far north of the equator, living on crops and domesticated animals for many generations. In the event of a drought or other natural catastrophe that caused crops to fail, milk and other dairy products might easily have become their primary source of calories. In times like these, the lactose-intolerant would become sick or malnourished. Since sick and malnourished individuals tend to have decreased fertility, lactose tolerance would be favored by natural selection. In other words, if these conditions persisted over enough time, eventually most, if not all, people would possess the ability to digest lactose because those who could not would not be making babies. None of this is to say that dairy is harmless, only that it is a reliable source of calories that appears to be able to sustain us through the ages of reproduction.

Most of the modern foods Paleo nutrition avoids have a much more cumulative affect than lactose intolerance. They may make us feel bad, but most people in the Western world have been eating them throughout their lives and have no idea that feeling better is an option. The important factor to our adaptation counterpoint, though, is that these harmful foods do not do enough damage early in life to negatively affect our reproductive fitness. So, if you want to think like your genes, eating as you have always eaten, having lots of kids at a young age, and then dropping dead at fifty is perfectly fine. There is nothing to adapt to in that story. But if you think like me, and I believe you do, fifty years is about halfway to the finish line.

## The Paleo Fad

It seems that every time someone in the media mentions Paleo, it is referred to as a fad diet. I realize that most of us believe the media to be all-knowing and infallible (sarcasm added at no additional cost to you!), but I think we should analyze these statements for truth anyway. If they are going to try to rob me of credibility, why not play the role of the heretic to the best of my ability?

Even if we leave out the couple of million years that our species was developing and talk only about anatomically modern *Homo sapiens*, we still have 200,000 years of hunting and gathering to discuss. To be more specific, if anatomically modern humans have been around for 200,000 years, and the agricultural revolution happened only approximately 10,000 years ago, we can confidently say that the Paleo diet reigned supreme and unabated for

190,000 years. Because there are still indigenous people hunting and gathering on the planet today, we can also say that Paleo has always been here, even before it gained the moniker "The Paleo Diet."

Wikipedia says, "A fad is any form of behavior that develops among a large population and is collectively followed with enthusiasm for some period, generally as a result of the behavior being perceived as novel in some way. A fad is said to 'catch on' when the number of people adopting it begins to increase rapidly. The behavior will normally fade quickly once the perception of novelty is gone."

Dictionary.com defines a fad as "a temporary fashion, notion, manner of conduct, etc., especially one followed enthusiastically by a group."

If we combine our knowledge of human hunting-and-gathering behavior with the above definitions of the word "fad," we easily arrive at two conclusions. First, if Paleo is a fad, it is the longest-running fad of all time. Second, those who call it a fad clearly do not understand even the most basic definition of Paleo and therefore should probably not be writing about it. But then again, I guess facts have never really been essential to the process of selling news or other products.

## This Is Not Dogma

I would like to make one quick point before we move on to my recommendations. As you now know, the Paleo concept grew out of the idea that natural selection has molded and shaped our biology. As such, Paleo is a lens through which we examine our nutrition, as well as other factors affecting our health, in an attempt to discover those inputs to which we are most adapted and avoid those that are harmful. All of this is fantastic and inconceivably valuable, but it is important to understand that not every step off the path has been bad, only that every step off the path is suspect. To put this another way, we should closely examine inputs and behavior that are very recent additions to human life, but we should not automatically vilify those things without good reason.

There are Paleo professionals who might disagree with some of the small details in this book. My views may be more or less restrictive than the views of others, and we all catch our fair share of flack from those with differing opinions, but we usually agree on the big picture. For me, the big picture is all about helping you, not wielding my Paleo knowledge against someone else's in a battle of the geeks, although I have learned a lot from such battles.

I have helped many more people than I could ever count using the information I'm sharing with you. Anecdotal? Yes. But still quite valuable to those who were helped. So, while I do believe I have the answers you seek, I am not the only player in the game. At various stages in your Paleo journey you may encounter other opinions regarding the minor details and those opinions could be worth a look. Science regularly brings us new information and we can expect it to continue doing so for a very long time. However, the basic foundational tenets of Paleo will never change. The foods we avoid are not coming back to the side of righteousness, and the foods we evolved to eat will never betray us. If anyone tries to convince you otherwise, he has an agenda based on something other than your health and fitness. Period.

# CHAPTER 7
# the right and wrong equipment

## Foods to Avoid

So, what *is* the natural diet for *Homo sapiens?* Let's start with what it is not. There have been many recent additions to our daily diet that have been particularly problematic. Removing just one of these offenders can sometimes have a dramatic affect on your health, but removing everything on the list is truly Paleo, and beneficial in magnificent and often unpredicted ways.

### Grains

Avoiding grains is definitely one of the defining principles of Paleo nutrition. Most people are astonished that we would ever want to avoid something that has been lauded as being so beneficial. When I talk to a new crowd about grains, I half expect someone to correct me by saying, "I think you mean *healthy whole grains.*" But in truth, grains have been a part of our diet only since the agricultural revolution, which means they are an intervention on our natural human nutrition. As I stated before, all deviations from the plan are not automatically a horrible sin against nature, but grains just happen to be big offenders.

To get to the root of the problem we have to ask, "Does this plant want to be eaten?" I know that sounds like an odd question, but plants are actually quite effective at avoiding being eaten. Some grow hard shells, sharp edges, or thorns. Some become bitter or poisonous. Some even cause sterility in the creatures that eat them. If a plant is being eaten it is probably either benefiting from the relationship, its reproductive capacity is unaffected, or it is still evolving its defenses against this particular offender. I'm sure there are exceptions, and I am not claiming to be a botanist, but these are basic rules of thumb. For an example of a mutually beneficial exchange, we need look no further than fruit. Fruit trees grow enticingly sweet fruits in which they hide their seeds. Creatures like monkeys, birds, and humans happen upon the tree's tasty offerings and carry the fruit away. When the valuable fruit flesh has been ingested, the seed is either discarded, like the pits of peaches and plums, or it is ingested and will be deposited later with a nice little starter supply of fertilizer. Either way, the tree has successfully sent its offspring to places it could not otherwise reach, since walking is out of the question.

Grains are grass seeds, and some birds, rodents, and insects are really the only animals that appear to be able to eat them without negative consequences. These seedeaters, or "granivores", have specialized digestive systems designed to extract nutrients from grains, like gizzards in birds, whereas grains must be milled for human consumption. If we do not mill grains, we are quite ineffective at digesting them, which would work out well for the plant because if the seeds are passed intact, we would have helped a grass procreate. This is also the relationship that grasses have with cows and other ruminants. The seeds usually survive digestion to be spread in the animal's droppings. Unfortunately for us, milling does not entirely sidestep the digestion issues. We are still left with lectins (plant proteins) and other anti-nutrients. Lectins are gut irritants in humans and most other mammals and they can really wreak havoc on the microvilli, or brush border, in our intestines.

Microvilli are amazing, hair-like microscopic protrusions on the inside walls of our intestines, and their job is to gather up nutrients from the flow of digestion to be absorbed into the bloodstream. But when lectins have their way with our microvilli, they increase our risk for a whole host of noninfectious diseases, especially autoimmune diseases, by causing a condition called *leaky gut* and by increasing systemic inflammation.

Leaky gut means that the tight junctions in the digestive wall have been damaged and particles have been allowed into the bloodstream that otherwise would be kept out. These particles, gram-negative bacteria for instance, are attacked by the immune system and destroyed. We can hope that our problems stop here, but it is quite possible that we are only getting started. When our immune systems kill invading particles, they create antibodies that charge around our bodies with little "Wanted" posters looking for the next particle that resembles the original invader. (OK, there may or may not be little "Wanted" posters, but the results are the same.) This arrangement works out great most of the time, but occasionally the invader will look enough like one of our own tissues to confuse the antibody. Enter autoimmunity.

Autoimmune diseases are conditions in which our immune systems are a little unclear about what is homegrown tissue and what is hostile interloper, and our antibodies attack parts we would rather keep intact and fully functional. Rheumatoid arthritis, Hashimoto's thyroiditis, lupus, Crohn's disease, psoriasis, and ulcerative colitis are, unfortunately, just a few of the many autoimmune diseases. There are also noninfectious diseases that are believed to be autoimmune in nature, like schizophrenia, multiple sclerosis, and narcolepsy. Some are considerably improved or eliminated by healing the gut, while others are chronic or even terminal. All are well worth avoiding, and eliminating grains from your diet will do the lion's share of the avoiding for you.

Another major problem with grains is the systemic inflammation caused by a constantly irritated gut. Systemic inflammation is basically an immune system that never quite makes it all the way back to a baseline state of rest. It is always a little bit too busy to simply relax and await the next intrusion. A busy immune system is one that has the potential to overlook a small part of its job now and then. As it turns out, one of the immune system's jobs is called apoptosis, which is programmed cell death, which occurs when cells are improperly replicated. If a bad cell is made and not destroyed through apoptosis, it may become a cancerous tumor. In reality, we all technically get the beginnings of cancer all the time, but our immune system wipes them out before they become a problem. Keeping your immune system constantly busy and overworked is flirting with disaster. I am by no means implicating grains as the sole cause of cancer, but since grains are major culprits in systemic inflammation and ubiquitous in our Western diet, it is not hard to see why cancer holds strong as a leading cause of death in the United States, second only to heart disease.

There is one more problem with grains worth mentioning. While grains do contain some of the minerals we need to be healthy, they also contain phytic acid, which binds to many of those minerals, making them useless to us. Fortified grains are basically a joke because if they were not fortified, their phytic acid content could actually leave us deficient in minerals like calcium, iron, and magnesium. It's funny that bread manufacturers use their labels to boast that their products are fortified when in reality fortifying is nothing more than an attempt to protect you from the damage their grains want to do to you. Nothing we are adapted to eat needs anything added to it to keep us safe.

Overall, grains are an excellent example of how interventions very often come with a hefty price tag. Everything was going fine with natural selection, and then one day we decide to change the rules as if we knew better than nature. Unfortunately, we don't make the rules, and while the rules may be bent they cannot be broken.

Here's the bottom line: Skip the grains. All grains. Trust me, you *will* feel better without them.

## Legumes

Legumes are beans and do not really warrant a huge discussion here because they cause many of the same gut-irritation issues that grains do except that they do their damage with chemical compounds called saponins instead of lectins. It is important to note that peanuts are actually legumes and not nuts. Legumes also tend to be a bit on the starchy side and therefore not a great choice for fat loss.

Here's the bottom line: Legumes are not that hard to avoid for most of us, so leave them out of your diet. Your gut will thank you.

## Vegetable Oils

Vegetable oils like corn, safflower, and soy are unnatural fats for humans, composed predominantly of linoleic acid, a highly unstable omega-6 polyunsaturated fatty acid (PUFA). The counterparts to omega-6 fatty acids in the human diet are omega-3 fatty acids, which include EPA (eicosapentaenoic acid) and DHA (docosahexaenoic acid), the valuable constituents in fish oil. If we still lived as hunter-gatherers, our omega-6 to omega-3 ratio would probably be around 2 to 1, but in the Standard American Diet the ratios are typically 15 to 1 or even higher. So, what's the big deal? As it turns out, omega-6 fatty acids are inflammatory, which means vegetable oils are in the same camp as grains when it comes to increasing systemic inflammation and risk of cancer.

Vegetable oils and the omega-6-to-omega-3 imbalance are also a culprit in loss of bone density. Osteoporosis and osteopenia are common today, especially among women. In typical fashion, the response of most "experts" is to simply throw more calcium at the bones instead of trying to find out why the bones might be losing density. Since calcium supplementation is downstream from the actual cause of the problem and may cause other problems, it makes a lot more sense to track down the real source of the problem. Vegetable oils appear to be a prime candidate for a good chunk of the blame.

Here's the bottom line: Avoid vegetable oils whenever possible. This may be tough when you eat out, but make the best of it by forgoing these rancid fats everywhere else in your life.

## Refined Sugar

Consumption of refined sugar is b-a-d, but you already knew that. If this is news to you, welcome back from Mars—a lot has changed while you were gone. You may especially enjoy the automobile and the telephone.

All joking aside, eating or drinking sugar increases glucose (blood sugar) levels to unnaturally high levels, and our bodies must compensate by producing unnaturally high levels of insulin. The problems associated with these conditions are many and quite common, including obesity, heart disease, type 2 diabetes, cancer, and Alzheimer's. We will discuss the basic physiology of sugar and excessive carbohydrate consumption shortly. Honey was the only sweetener available in the Paleolithic period, so feel free to eat all the honey you want, but only after you get stung by ten bees per serving. Of course I am joking again. Do not go looking for bees to sting you. More on honey and other sugar substitutes later.

Few things in our modern diet spark as much emotion as sugar. When people say they love their favorite sugar-laden treat, you can almost see the truth of their words in their eyes. We don't generally eat sweets because we're hungry, and nobody believes they're harmless, but they are ever so enticing. Reread the Taste and Flavor section (page 51) to remind yourself why sugar should be avoided.

Here's the bottom line: Break up with sugar. Your relationship is dysfunctional anyway.

## High-Fructose Corn Syrup

High-fructose corn syrup is one of those substances in the human diet that riles me up the most. First the facts, then the rant. Fructose is basically a bad sugar for humans. Upon ingestion, fructose is shuttled through the hepatic portal vein to the liver, where it is either converted to glycogen, the stored form of glucose, or to triglycerides for storage in your fat cells. It is not immediately used by the cells for energy. When we find fructose in nature, we inevitably also find fiber, as in fruit, which slows down the absorption of fructose and at least makes it a little less problematic. I don't want to vilify fructose entirely because in natural doses it is probably fine for healthy people, but fructose is often found in completely unnatural doses in the Western diet, mostly because of high-fructose corn syrup. Sucrose, or table sugar, is 50 percent glucose and 50 percent fructose, but high-fructose corn syrup is only 45 percent glucose and 55 percent fructose. That slight change in composition is enough to cause it to be processed by the body like ethanol alcohol, the stuff that puts the "adult" in adult beverages, which leads to the same kinds of problems that alcohol causes in the liver. Thus, consuming high-fructose corn syrup in the myriad processed foods it is used in can also mean a huge increase in disorders like hepatic steatosis (nonalcoholic fatty-liver disease) and obesity.

Now, for some unabashed grumpiness. When was the last time you were out and about and saw a child drinking a soft drink? Can you be certain that the memory you are recalling now is actually the most recent time you were aware of a child drinking a soda in public? Probably not. Kids drinking soft drinks are such a common sight that most of us would not even process the sight as a memory. But what if that kid were drinking vodka out of a flask? You would be appalled, right? You might even take steps to make sure his parents paid for such neglect. Why? People do not tend to die from getting drunk unless there is an accident involved. We can be reasonably sure that this child and his flask would not end up behind the wheel of a car, but he could theoretically fall down some stairs or pass out on his back and drown in his own vomit, rock-star style. Let's be honest, though. The big worry for alcoholics is liver disease, which can be caused quite adequately by ingesting large quantities of high-fructose corn syrup. Why, then, is it completely fine for a child to guzzle soda laden with high-fructose corn syrup?

Here's the bottom line: Get grumpy with me and commit to deleting high-fructose corn syrup from your diet and the diet of your kids as well.

## Artificial Sweeteners and Sugar Substitutes

For the real problems behind artificial sweeteners and sugar substitutes, you will need to remember the discussion on taste and flavor and the addictive quality of highly palatable, low-nutrition foods. Once you understand those basics, you could probably figure out for yourself why sugar replacements are no good, but let's take a look at a few of the details anyway.

I do not think I have ever delivered a seminar without at least one person asking about an artificial sweetener. My answer: They are all bad, all the time. Yes, there appears to be some small amount of data that says stevia may be OK, but I don't care. The reason I remain unconvinced is that the systems I mentioned in the Taste and Flavor section are broken by artificial sweeteners, just as they are by junk food. Even if an artificial sweetener is harmless biochemically (which would be rare), increasing palatability without increasing nutritional value is not a great recipe for health, and I firmly believe that the science will eventually back me up on this. I will not rehash all the science here, but I hope to appeal to you logically. After everything I threw at you regarding flavor and dopamine, it should not be difficult to see that when you add flavor, and therefore increase food reward, you are playing with fire. Even adding artificial sweeteners to Paleo-approved foods may still cause trouble because increased palatability means increased odds of overeating. Regularly stuffing yourself to the gills, even with healthy foods, will probably mean fat gain.

Honey was available in various locales around the world in the late Paleolithic, and is still available to many of the hunter-gatherers living today. Frank W. Marlowe, in his insightful book *The Hadza: Hunter-Gatherers of Tanzania*, has this to say about the Hadza and honey collecting:

*When men are out on walkabout, they always have their bows and arrows, but they often stop at trees to check on beehives. They can tell by watching the bees whether there is much honey ready to harvest. A man often puts his ear to the trunk to listen to the bees. After monitoring trees in the area around their camp, they may decide that it is time to raid the hives, and then they carry their axes (in addition to their bows). If they should see game worth pursuit, they abandon the search for honey and pursue the animal until they kill it or it gets away. Honey collecting does not pose a substantial tradeoff with hunting.*

I find it interesting that while the Hadza do forage for honey, they still place more value on meat. We, on the other hand, will trade our souls and our first-born children for sweets. Honey is sugar. Don't fool yourself into believing that it is harmless. Same thing with maple syrup.

Agave nectar is another sugar substitute that has become popular in recent years. It was touted as being healthier than sugar, but in reality it is almost entirely fructose. Go back to the previous section on high-fructose corn syrup for all the fun to be had with agave nectar.

In regards to avoiding artificial sweeteners and sugar substitutes, my best advice is to go cold turkey. For example, if you *need* to add something to your coffee, try switching to only heavy cream. I bet you will adapt to the change in flavor in a day or two.

As I said before, you should not have to choke down flavorless foods, and you should enjoy eating, but falling in love with the flavor of the wrong foods can keep your health and fitness goals out of reach.

## Soy

Soy was not considered a food in the United States until the 1920s, and it is nasty stuff indeed. To begin with, soy contains a substantial amount of saponins, those mean, little gut irritants found in all legumes. Good gut health is essential to avoiding autoimmune diseases and reducing systemic inflammation. But soy is even worse than other legumes when it comes to hostile behavior because it is a potent source of phytoestrogens. Phytoestrogens mimic estrogen in our bodies. Estrogen is a powerful hormone with multiple jobs and should not to be trifled with.

Soy consumption has been linked to thyroid issues, cancer, heart disease, and reproductive issues, among other problems. To my knowledge, these links are all only correlations at this point, but I would hate to be one of the statistics that led to better research nailing soy as the cause of one of them. Because smaller bodies are more affected by soy, it should not be used in infant formulas. Unfortunately, soy formula is popular and recommended by many "experts."

Here's the bottom line: Avoid soy as if it were toxic, because it is.

## Most Dairy

Dairy is a tricky subject for me. I would love to tell everyone to avoid all dairy all the time, but the data does not back me up as well as I would like it to. I believe that milk is always a bad idea for everyone. The primary protein in milk is casein. Casein is tough for humans to digest and may even promote cancer, although I haven't seen any clear data on that subject. It should also be crystal clear to anyone who thinks about it that milk is a growth promoter. The main purpose of milk is to turn a small mammal into a big mammal in a very short time. When we look at the chemical makeup of milk, we do in fact find growth promoters such as insulin-like growth factor 1 (IGF-1). Anything that promotes growth could be a cancer risk because more cellular reproduction means more chance for errors, thus more chance of the formation of cancerous cells. Picture the *I Love Lucy* episode where Lucy is in the chocolate factory when you think of your immune system: The conveyor belt is moving so fast that your immune system may not be able to keep up, which might mean that badly reproduced cells are not properly disposed of through apoptosis.

*But*, it appears that fermented forms of dairy are less offensive, and possibly much less offensive. Fermentation can break down much of the casein, kind of like partial digestion. The growth promoters can be destroyed in the same way. Therefore, fermented dairy products, like yogurt, cheese, cottage cheese, and sour cream, *may* not be problematic.

There are two exceptions in the world of dairy. Pastured butter and heavy cream are fine for most people and can be a healthy addition to your Paleo diet, provided you do not suffer from any autoimmune disorders. Both butter and heavy cream are formed from almost entirely healthy animal fats. Be aware of the caloric density of butter and heavy cream, though. Consuming large quantities of either can make for difficult fat loss, but don't worry about it too much unless you intend to down a bowl of butter and a glass of heavy cream. Adding butter and/or cream to recipes will be fine for almost everyone. Some people will feel better with the removal of butter and heavy cream, so some experimentation may be in order, but this is not a first order of business. Unless you suffer an autoimmune disorder, reasonable quantities of butter and heavy cream are generally fine in the beginning of your transition to Paleo and can be revisited when everything else is dialed in. Those who are lactose-intolerant may have trouble with heavy cream, but most will be fine with butter.

Here's the bottom line: Avoid dairy if you want to be really healthy, and especially if your goal is fat loss. If you do consume it from time to time, try to buy only pastured and well-fermented dairy, like Greek-style yogurt made from raw milk from grass-fed cows. Again, avoidance is better.

# *Foods to Enjoy*

The following foods are the heart and soul of Paleo eating and our best attempt at recreating the diet and robust health of our ancient ancestors. If you have been eating a typical Western diet for a long time, these are the foods that will bring you renewed vitality and the energy to love being alive.

## Meat

Meat, and red meat in particular, is the cornerstone of Paleo nutrition and the reason we became the humans we are today. That great, big brain you are using right now to process the information in this book is a direct result of your ancient ancestors eating lots of meat. Meat is a dense source of nutrients, and more meat consumption by our forebearers allowed for the shrinking of our digestive systems and the growth of our brains. We now have isotopic bone analyses that definitively show meat to have been a primary source of calories throughout *Homo sapien* history. I'm sure I'm breaking a few hearts, but vegetarianism and veganism did not exist prior to the last couple of thousand years.

Since breaking the rules is what got us into all our modern health troubles, and returning to the basics is the way back out, meat must return to its place of prominence in our diets if we desire peak health and fitness. But it is also important to consider the lives and health of the animals we eat. The best meat will come from animals that lived the way nature intended them to live. For example, cows eat grass, not corn and other grains. When they are forced to eat corn and grains on factory feedlots, the fatty-acid profile in their fat changes, and their otherwise healthy fat becomes pro-inflammatory in our digestive systems.

Pork and fowl have fatty-acid profiles that are not quite as favorable as those of beef, and people whose diets consist primarily of pork and fowl will probably suffer a little more systemic inflammation than those who eat more red meat. I know this is a bummer for you if you are not a red meat fan, because you were probably thinking you could just eat a lot of chicken. Unfortunately, this is not how you evolved. That said, a diet composed of very little red meat, but in which meat of some kind is still the bulk of caloric intake, is vastly superior to a typical Western diet.

Organ meats are some of the most nutrient-dense foods in the human diet. In fact, organ meats are prized by hunter-gatherers, with the muscle (which we favor today) usually eaten after the organ meat is gone. Few foods in our modern diet offer the vitamin and mineral profile of beef liver. Unfortunately, offal (organ meat) is not popular in Western cuisine, and many of us have not had enough exposure to liver, kidneys, heart, and the like to acquire a taste for them. If you absolutely hate organ meats, I will not force them on you, but please promise to at least give them another go. At least research your recipe options for grass-fed beef liver, and see if you can find one that sounds palatable. It's worth the effort and experimentation to add a food to your diet that has unbeatable nutritional value.

Pet-peeve time. Meat is defined as "animal flesh that is eaten as food." Last time I checked, fish and shellfish were members of the animal kingdom. Therefore, saying "meat and seafood" is like saying "animals and fish." Fish and shellfish are meat and both are highly recommended additions to your diet. Cold-water fish, like salmon and tuna, are excellent sources of quality fats, but all fish and shellfish are great. Try to find wild-caught fish whenever possible because farmed fish is like feedlot cattle: when we feed them garbage and confine them to inhumanely small spaces, their meat is less nourishing and sometimes problematic.

Eggs are also among the foods of the gods, and since they are animals-to-be, we will include them with meat. Chicken eggs, duck eggs, goose eggs, ostrich eggs, and virtually every other bird's eggs you can get your hands on are great. OK, California condor eggs are a bad choice, but any bird not on the endangered list is fair game. Be sure to eat the entire egg. Throwing out the yolk makes the whole act pointless. If you are worried about cholesterol, keep reading. If you suffer from an autoimmune disorder, try removing eggs from your diet for at least a month and see how you feel. Eggs contain a few proteins that could pose a problem in the gut, increasing permeability and leading to autoimmune issues.

Here's the bottom line: Make meat your primary source of calories, and try to eat it at every meal. The bulk of your meat should come from pastured ruminants (red meat).

## Vegetables

Vegetables are great sources of many vitamins and minerals, and they can be eaten at every meal, but they should not replace meat as your primary source of calories over an extended period of time. In other words, it's OK to have the occasional salad without meat, but you should not look back at a week of meals and find more total calories consumed from vegetables than from meat.

A wide variety of vegetables are available to most of us, but we often tend to get stuck eating the same four or five veggies all the time. Make an effort to eat as many different types of vegetables as possible. Fibrous vegetables—like broccoli, spinach, kale, and cauliflower—are best for fat loss, while starchy vegetables, like sweet potatoes and butternut squash, can stall fat-loss goals.

If you suffer from an autoimmune disease, avoid nightshades. "Nightshade" is the common name for any plant in the family Solanaceae, which includes tomatoes, eggplants, peppers, and potatoes (but not sweet potatoes). Nightshades can cause gut permeability, but they are probably OK for people with healthy digestion and no autoimmune issues.

I realize that some readers may be thinking, "If I don't eat a pile of vegetables as high as my waist each day, where will I get my vitamins and minerals?" Interestingly, we do not tend to see deficiencies in those cultures, like the Inuits, still eating their traditional diet and consuming almost no vegetables at all. Looking a little closer, we find that vitamin and mineral deficiencies are not always about low consumption but are more often about misuse of the vitamins and minerals that are consumed. We see the same thing with vitamin C in diets consisting of too many processed carbohydrates. Glucose (blood sugar) and vitamin C both require insulin to enter our cells. The problem is that glucose gets preferential treatment. Thus, when the Standard American Diet results in high levels of glucose it also results in a lot of wasted vitamin C. This relationship of glucose and vitamin C is called glucose-ascorbate antagonism (GAA).

None of this is to say that vegetables are useless, unhealthy, or should not be eaten. Vegetables are an important part of Paleo nutrition, but not more important than meat.

Here's the bottom line: Eat vegetables every day, but if you leave anything on your plate, make it veggies and not meat.

## Fruit

Fruit is yummy. It is kind of like plant candy. Healthy people can treat fruit as they would vegetables: fruit is great, but it should not replace meat as your prime source of calories. Most fruits, like veggies, are loaded with vitamins and minerals that can contribute to health.

However, fruit comes with a caveat. You may have noticed that I said "healthy people" in the preceding paragraph, and while most people in the Western world might be considered *normal*, most are not truly healthy.

Fructose, a.k.a. *fruit sugar*, plays a big role in those sweet fruit flavors we all love. As discussed in the section on high-fructose corn syrup (see page 86), fructose is not the most human-friendly sugar. Enter agricultural selection and things can get a little sketchy for fruit.

Let's say we wind the clock back 10,000 years and you plant the first two apple seeds ever planted by a human. The trees grow, making you the first apple farmer on earth. Since these first two trees provided easy calories for you and your family, you decide to repeat the process by planting more seeds. One of your original two trees grew sweeter apples, but you are just getting the hang of this farming thing so you plant seeds from both trees. When you realized that the seeds from the tree that grew the sweeter apples produced offspring that also grew sweeter apples, you opted to only plant seeds from the sweetest apple trees. Rinse and repeat for 10,000 years back to the present and we have apples that are much sweeter than any apple found anywhere in nature because we have agriculturally selected them to be as sweet as possible. *As sweet as possible* means *a bunch more fructose.*

Consuming copious quantities of the sweetest fruits isn't the best idea for most people, but anyone with an aggressive fat-loss goal or a metabolic disorder, like insulin resistance, should consider limiting fruit, or maybe even eliminating it entirely. Some people find that seasonal fruit consumption works well once they are healthy, which means: get your fruit from a local source, like a farmer's market, to be sure you are eating fruit in the season it is naturally available in your area.

In my opinion, fruit juice should never be consumed by anyone, ever. Juice is basically pure bad stuff. We will talk more about juice when we come to liquid food.

Here's the bottom line: Fruit is for healthy people, and should be eaten responsibly.

## The Maybe List

There are a few modern foods that are not technically Paleo-approved but do warrant some discussion. Please note that I am covering this topic because I'm an honest person. I would love to lie and tell you that borderline or questionable foods should never be consumed, but I trust you and I believe you will make responsible decisions.

## We Covered These Two Already ...

But I'll mention them again: fermented dairy products and fruit. Fermented dairy products are "maybes" because while fermentation may assist in breaking down casein, lactose, and growth promoters (see page 89), the jury is still out on whether that is beneficial enough to warrant consuming these products. Fruits are "maybes" because some can be high in fructose. Those who have the strongest desire to get healthy and fit as fast as possible should abstain from all dairy (except maybe butter and heavy cream, in responsible quantities) and all fruit, at least until they reach their goals.

## Nuts and Seeds

Nuts have a place in Paleo, but there are a couple of things you should know. First, most nuts are a little high in omega-6 polyunsaturated fatty acids. These are the pro-inflammatory fats that are the major problem with vegetable oils. Since it can sometimes be tough to entirely avoid vegetable oils, especially if you eat out a lot, it is important to keep your omega-6 intake as low as possible whenever you can. Fortunately, we don't tend to sit down to a meal of nuts; leaving them out is a step in the right direction in terms of limiting inflammation.

The other concern with nuts is their phytic acid content. Phytic acid is the antinutrient also found in grains that steals minerals from us. Again, it may not be that big of a deal because we do not usually eat a plate of nuts for dinner, but snackers beware. I am not a big fan of snacking anyway, especially for fat loss. More on that subject later.

Here's the bottom line: A handful of nuts each day is probably fine for most people, but try not to go overboard. That is all you really need to know about nuts ... in a nutshell. (Sorry, I couldn't resist.)

## Alcohol

I would have to be a naïve moron to think that none of you will ever touch another drop of alcohol. And, rest assured, I'm not asking anyone to live like a monk in a mountaintop abbey. A little alcohol consumption might even be healthy, but even if it isn't, most of us are going to have a few more drinks between here and the grave.

But alcohol consumption can be particularly disadvantageous to anyone attempting to lose fat because it is all empty calories, totally bereft of nutritional value. While calories are not the sole factor involved in fat gain or loss, they do technically still count, and everything we eat or drink should be promoting health. Give this concept some thought when presented with an opportunity to have a drink. As long as you weigh your alcohol consumption against your desire to be fit and healthy, nobody can tell you what is right for you. But mindlessly drinking yourself into a stupor just because it's Friday should mean that you have decided to accept the state of your body.

Red wine is probably the best choice, but moderation is the key. A glass per day may be OK for most people who aren't aiming to lose fat. To clarify, a glass is about five ounces, so don't go thinking you can pour your wine into that fishbowl you drank a margarita out of last Cinco de Mayo and call it a glass. If you prefer hard alcohol, try to avoid the fruity-sweet concoctions that always make you feel like death warmed over the next morning. Beer is a bad idea unless it's gluten-free, which makes it a little less bad. Unfortunately, good gluten-free beer can cost more than twice as much as regular beer. I know I just crushed a few beer drinkers, but it had to be said.

Here's the bottom line: To quote Robb Wolf, "Drink to the degree that it does not negatively affect the way you look, feel, and perform, but it positively enhances your sex life." (I always tell my wife that the more she drinks, the better I look. Consequently she is a blazing drunk, and I appreciate the effort.)

## Caffeine

I have always found the subject of caffeine a little amusing. Critics say caffeine is the path to an early grave. Proponents say caffeine is a miracle that helps you burn fat and is good for your brain. But when all is said and done, the data can be a little tenuous on both sides of the argument. I have yet to see a study that proved caffeine was either terrible or amazing. There are studies suggesting that caffeine may be a little unhealthy, and there are studies appearing to show some small benefit to caffeine consumption, but no earth-shattering results on either side. As with all science, there may be research some day proving caffeine absolutely evil or absolutely benign or absolutely beneficial, and I reserve the right to change my mind about caffeine when any of those days come. Meanwhile, though, I enjoy my coffee in moderation, and I have never experienced any ill effects in myself personally or in any client when caffeine was consumed *responsibly*. Which brings me to an important point.

In my professional opinion, caffeine is for people who have good metabolic health. When we consume caffeine we are basically borrowing energy from our adrenals. You can ask too much of your adrenals, but this will probably not happen as a result of simply drinking coffee unless you guzzle espresso all the livelong day. That said, taking into consideration other factors that may affect metabolic health, a great many people should be careful with caffeine.

If you sleep poorly, caffeine is not a great idea for you, even though you probably think you need it to get through a day after not-enough sleep. Caffeine may or may not be causing or worsening your sleep problems, but it's best to address them from a caffeine-free vantage point. Have you noticed that an amount of caffeine that used to get you wired now only sustains you? This is not because you have settled into a nice groove; it is because you are trying to treat your lack of energy with an exogenous substance and are building up a tolerance to your "medicine." Eventually you may find yourself in a place where mostly harmless caffeine becomes harmful. Also, if you are stressed out, insulin-resistant, fatigued, or a cardio addict, you should think about eliminating, or at least reducing, caffeine until you get healthy: You are not actually fixing your lack of energy with caffeine, and in conjunction with those other variable, may be making things worse.

Regardless of your goals, there are few ways to get your shot of caffeine without sacrificing your health. Coffee and tea are reasonable methods of caffeine delivery, but not if they are loaded with sugar (including flavored syrup) before you can choke them down. And you shouldn't ever touch energy drinks.

If you're wondering about how caffeine affects you, take a break from it for a week or two to see how you feel. The first couple of days might be rough, but if you end up feeling great, you can assume that caffeine is a problem for you and should be avoided or reintroduced carefully.

Here's the bottom line: Assess your sleep patterns, energy level, and overall health. If everything seems pretty good, responsible caffeine consumption is probably OK for you, but you might consider taking a break from it to be sure.

# CHAPTER 8

# good fundamentals
# for the win

## OK, OK, We Can Talk About
## Macronutrients for a Minute

Brace yourself, what I am going to say next may come as a shock to you. *Humans evolved to eat food.* I know—crazy, right? Listening to "common knowledge" you would think that we were supposed to be eating carbs, fat, protein, vitamins, and minerals, and the fact that they are combined into something we recognize as food is incidental.

As insane as I must sound right now, I want you to get those old ideas out of your head posthaste. Macronutrients (carbohydrate, fat, and protein) can be a topic of conversation when we tweak the knobs and dials for specific goals, but this stuff falls into place for almost everyone when we swap modern processed food for Paleo-approved human food. The vast majority of people eating Paleo will never need to weigh and measure anything. There is simply no need to make such a big fuss about it. Nonetheless, we need to touch on each of the macronutrients so you will understand the big picture. I will try not to get too scientific.

### Fat

Did you shudder when you read the title of this section? If so, you are not alone. Fat, especially saturated animal fat, has been vilified in the medical community and media for decades. It seems rational to associate dietary fat with the stored fat on our buns and thighs, but in reality our excess body fat is mostly due to processed-carbohydrate consumption, which we will discuss soon.

Indeed, it is true that some fats are bad. We covered vegetable oils already, but we also need to throw man-made trans fats in there with the bad guys. Trans fats are also called "partially hydrogenated" or "hydrogenated fats" on labels. If you encounter a food containing trans fat, set it back down and walk away. For years we were told that these nasty, little chemistry experiments were fine, and that foods containing trans fats were better for us that those that contained saturated fat. If you are older than twenty, at some point you probably purchased margarine to avoid the saturated fat in butter. Today, most of us have learned that trans fats are indeed nasty. Animal research has shown that trans fats cause more total weight gain per calorie consumed, and they are also associated with inflammation and heart disease. Fortunately, a solid Paleo diet avoids trans fats by accident because only processed foods contain these artificially altered aberrations.

The big deal with saturated fat is the common belief that it is the evil villain behind heart disease. The story, often called the Cholesterol or Lipid Hypothesis, goes like this:

*When we eat fat, our cholesterol level goes up and cholesterol clogs our arteries, causing heart disease.*

If that was your first time hearing this hypothesis, you have somehow avoided all media and interaction with other humans since the 1970s. The problem with this widespread dogma is that it is completely wrong. Good science has proved time and time again that neither saturated fat nor total cholesterol levels are in any way related to heart disease. There do not even appear to be any loose correlations.

In 2010, a paper was published in the *American Journal of Clinical Nutrition* titled "Meta-analysis of Prospective Cohort Studies Evaluating the Association of Saturated Fat with Cardiovascular Disease." A meta-analysis is an evaluation of the data and results of multiple related studies. The idea is to get a bigger picture by looking at a lot of relevant data at one time. These researchers looked at twenty-one studies and found the following:

*A meta-analysis of prospective epidemiologic studies showed that there is no significant evidence for concluding that dietary saturated fat is associated with an increased risk of CHD (coronary heart disease) or CVD (cardiovascular disease). More data are needed to elucidate whether CVD risks are likely to be influenced by the specific nutrients used to replace saturated fat.*

This is but one study among very many, and many doctors and scientists have tackled this ridiculousness. It is actually an easy task to find inconsistencies that punch holes in the cholesterol-lipid hypothesis. For example, the French eat a lot more fat than we do here in the U.S., but they suffer much less heart disease. Also, the Australian Aboriginals suffer from perhaps the highest rate of heart disease in the world, yet their cholesterol levels are very low. In real science, information like this would lead to a lot more research. In the pseudo science necessary to push lots of drugs onto the market and into consumers, inconsistencies are simply called "paradoxes" and subsequently ignored forever.

In reality, saturated animal fats have sustained us for as long as we have been on this planet. They are excellent sources of energy that are relatively benign regarding our health. Fatty acids in general are also essential for a healthy brain and central nervous system, and low-fat diets are strongly correlated to depression and anxiety. Your brain is made up of fats like DHA (Docosahexaenoic acid), EPA (Eicosapentaenoic acid), Arachidonic acid, and Phosphatidylserine. No need to memorize those—there won't be a test. Just remember that your brain likes fat.

I could write a hundred pages about fatty acids alone, but I'd probably lose you! If you want to go further by yourself, I highly recommend *The Great Cholesterol Con,* by Dr. Malcolm Kendrick, but he is by no means the only soldier in this fight. Tom Naughton, in his wonderful documentary *Fat Head,* does an outstanding job of telling the story of how we got to where we are today despite a complete lack of scientific data to support our current beliefs concerning fat and cholesterol. Gary Taubes wrote an exhaustive exploration of heart disease and obesity titled *Good Calories, Bad Calories.* It can be a tough read, but well worth it. Taubes also wrote an article for the *New York Times* titled "What if It's All Been a Big Fat Lie"? which tackled much of what we think we know about fat. The article ran back in 2002, but nothing changed.

If you harbor a fear of fat, you are a victim of bad science. If you do not want to take my word for it, please do some research. I have given you a few great places to start. My only hope is that you will change your perspective. Start reading—your health depends on it.

## Protein

Protein is the stuff our tissues are made of. Which means that increasing muscle mass and gaining strength requires it. And unless you are a massive body builder already, more muscle is an essential part of getting fit and healthy—even if your goal is fat loss. More on that subject to come.

All proteins are made up of amino acids, sometimes called "the building blocks of protein." There are twenty-one amino acids that we need concern ourselves with, of which nine are essential, meaning that our bodies cannot synthesize them. Lysine and tryptophan are not usually found throughout the plant world in the high concentrations that they are found in the meat world; vegetarians and vegans have to plan carefully to get enough of them through whole foods or take supplements. The other seven essential amino acids are leucine, isoleucine, valine, methionine, phenylalanine, threonine, and histidine.

The average person needs between 70 and 100 grams of protein per day. A good rule of thumb is approximately 0.8 grams of protein per pound of lean body mass to stay healthy and fit. That translates to 75 grams of protein for a 125-pound woman with 25 percent body fat. Fortunately, there is really no need for most of us to get out the calculator. Just make meat the main source of calories in most of your meals and you will be fine. In other words, going Paleo is all it takes.

## Carbohydrate

Believe it or not, there is no such thing as an essential carbohydrate. Which is to say that you could live the rest of your life without eating another gram of carbohydrate and never be the worse for it. Some Eskimos still living traditionally come very close to zero carbohydrate consumption in a year. An observation study often cited in the Paleo community consisted of the explorers Vilhjalmur Stefansson and Karsten Anderson spending a year beginning in 1928 at Bellevue Hospital in New York City eating a diet of nothing but meat. They claimed to have eaten this way in good health while living with the Eskimos in the Arctic. At the end of the yearlong study, and after much testing, both men had lost a little weight, despite eating between 2,000 and 3,100 calories of meat per day, and all their health markers, including cholesterol, were either improved or unaffected.

I am not saying to avoid carbohydrates entirely, or that carbs are evil, but it is telling that we do not actually *need* them. The unnatural quantities of carbohydrates in our processed modern foods are destroying our health. Let's take a closer look at the problems we encounter when we eat carbohydrates in forms and quantities that our bodies do not comprehend.

# Insulin and Fat Storage

Brace yourself: I'm about to get a little science-y. A quick primer in some basic physiology is necessary to help you understand why it is important to eat in a way that makes sense to your body. This information is particularly valuable if your goal is fat loss, but it is valuable to everyone, so hang on. I have kept it brief and highly oversimplified, but I think you will get the gist. Let me begin with a caveat: If you get to the other side of the next two sections and you don't quite get it all, it's not a big deal—some people thrive on lots of information, some don't. OK, here we go.

Let's assume that you have soaked up every word I've written so far and haven't made any changes yet. Maybe you are making an effort to lose weight, but you are still "doing" diets instead of eating like a human. Your head is still full of myths and wives' tales. Your typical day of eating probably looks something like this:

- Oatmeal and whole wheat toast for breakfast
- Fat-free sugar-laden coffee drink to get you over your midmorning slump
- Subway sandwich for lunch because Jared lost weight that way
- A bagel, granola bar, or other processed carbs to get you over the afternoon slump
- Pasta for dinner
- Something crunchy or sweet between 8 and 10 p.m.

Overall, it was a low-fat day, and since *everyone knows* that fat is what makes us fat, you feel pretty good about your efforts. You take solace in the fact that the entire nation has been eating like this for decades. There is really no need to assume that these food choices could be the problem, right? Well, as you are now beginning to learn, we are not getting off scott free.

Here's the inside scoop: Carbohydrates are converted to glucose (blood sugar), so each of these meals/snacks causes a hefty dose of glucose to enter your bloodstream very quickly. Your body closely regulates glucose to keep it within a safe range—not too high and not too low. After you consume easily digestible carbohydrates like the ones on your menu above, your pancreas must secrete insulin to mitigate the resulting elevated glucose. One of insulin's primary jobs is to feed the glucose in your bloodstream to hungry cells so they can use it for energy. Then the leftover glucose is sent to the liver to be turned into triglycerides for storage in your fat cells. Are you still with me? Take a deep breath. OK, let's keep moving.

The story so far: Carbs are eaten and broken down into glucose, insulin sends glucose to your cells to be used as energy or to the liver to be turned into triglycerides that will be stored as fat on your buns and thighs. Make note of this transformation from whole wheat toast to stored body fat.

Moving on. Your Standard American Diet (SAD) keeps glucose and insulin high throughout your day thanks to all those processed carbs. This can eventually lead to *insulin resistance* in those cells that use glucose as energy. Insulin resistance is when insulin is ever present and its "I come bearing food" signal to the cells is reduced to a whisper and then finally ignored. This causes your pancreas to produce more insulin to get the same job done, and this in turn keeps insulin ever-present in ever-greater quantities. If you are still with me, you'll realize that you are amassing more and more insulin in your bloodstream.

Hyperinsulinemia, this state of elevated insulin, is bad. Very bad. Robb Wolf once suggested if you Google "hyperinsulinemia" and any noninfectious disease that comes to mind, you will find strong correlations in more links than you would ever take the time to read. When insulin hangs around too often, it also means that you store a lot of fat and have trouble using fat as energy. This is because insulin is your body's primary storage hormone. Here's how it works (take another deep breath).

High levels of glucose in the bloodstream are toxic: Just ask a type 1 diabetic. As I just said, your body devotes a lot of energy to keeping glucose within a fairly tight range. This means that glucose is used for energy before fatty acids because glucose cannot be allowed to hang out in the blood and cause problems. You can store only a small amount of glucose (as glycogen) in your liver and muscles, but a nearly unlimited amount of fat can be stored. This is why the liver converts the extra glucose to triglycerides and ships it off for storage in the fat cells—toxicity problem solved, and energy is stored for later.

Hang in there—I'm getting to the juicy part. At the fat cell, an enzyme called lipoprotein lipase (LPL) acts as the doorman, ushering fatty acids into the fat cells. Inside the fat cell, another enzyme, hormone-sensitive lipase (HSL), has the job of cleaving the first sulfide bond on the triglycerides and releasing fatty acids to be used as energy. So, LPL is working when you are storing fat, and HSL is working when you are burning fat. Here's the rub: Both of these enzymes are sensitive to insulin. When insulin is present, LPL is on duty and is storing more fat in your fat cells. When insulin isn't present, HSL is on duty and you are using your stored fat as energy.

If you have been following me, this process will make perfect sense. Since we know that glucose cannot be allowed to hang out and must be used first, we also know that there is no reason to access stored fat in the presence of glucose and, therefore, insulin. When insulin is in the bloodstream, the message is clear: Get rid of glucose before using stored fat. Now it is easy to see why hyperinsulinemia and insulin resistance are a problem. They keep you in fat-storage mode, without the ability to access your stored fat for energy, for long enough to make you plump and squishy.

I am not trying to paint carbohydrates and insulin as villains. They are a normal and natural part of human nutrition and biochemistry. What is not normal is our mass consumption of processed carbohydrates, both in unnatural forms and in never-ending supply regardless of season. A solid Paleo diet, *along with proper exercise*, will make you healthier and leaner by allowing you to become insulin sensitive again and helping you re-adapt to using stored fat as energy so your fat cells can go back to being the batteries they are supposed to be instead of the warehouses they have become.

## Cravings

Now that we have a basic understanding of insulin and how we store fat, let's tackle the science behind cravings.

Remember the last time you lost control and ate something you later regretted? This is probably going to happen again as your body adjusts to healthy eating and you loosen the hold an unnaturally high carbohydrate intake has had on you. You might be cruising through your day, minding your business, and find yourself completely overcome with cravings. It might be all you can do to think about anything but whatever crunchy or sweet indulgence is in closest proximity to you. Whatever or whoever lies between you and the nearest pile of processed carbohydrates will be at risk of being trampled to death. What the heck is that all about?

It's all about our new-old friends glucose and insulin. If your daily diet has looked something like the one on page 102 for most of your adult life, your body has become highly adapted to using glucose for energy while storing fat. Lipoprotein lipase (LPL) has constantly been on duty ushering fatty acids into your fat cells, and hormone-sensitive lipase (HSL) has been pretty much sitting on the bench instead of releasing fat from your fat cells. Ah, yes, there can be a downside to being a highly adaptive creature. After years of this eating behavior, your body thinks this is the new normal, and it's not about to let you change the rules without a fight!

Let's be clear, however: You are not *fat adapted*. Rather, you lack *metabolic flexibility*. In other words, your body does not readily release stored energy (fat) from your batteries (fat cells) and use it to run your generators (mitochondria), and your mitochondria are inefficient at using fat for energy because they are *waaaay* out of practice. You have been pumping a constant supply of glucose (from processed carbs) into your bloodstream, and since glucose must be used first, your fat cells have turned into warehouses instead of batteries. To correct this, your fat cells must release fatty acids, and your mitochondria must accept those long-lost friends as fuel. This might take a while. You didn't get into your current state overnight, and you're not going to get out of it with just a flip of the switch.

As we discussed before, when you eat a processed-carb-laden meal, you get a nice spike in glucose, your pancreas kicks out a bunch of insulin to mitigate the glucose, and the glucose is fed to your hungry cells, stored as glycogen, or turned into fat and stuffed into your buns and thighs. When the glucose is all gone, a healthy body shifts into fat-burning mode and uses the fat it just stored to keep on trucking. But your body can't remember how to make the shift. Glucose is all it really knows. That leaves just one option: Scream for more glucose! Cravings are otherwise known as screams for more glucose.

There is an easy way to distinguish cravings from hunger. Simply swap out the food you are craving for something Paleo-approved. If you are truly hungry, most foods will sound good. I've said it more times than I can count: Nobody ever loses his cool at ten o'clock at night and eats a pound of broccoli or a twenty-ounce steak. The reality of cravings is more like, "Where did this empty ice cream carton come from, and why is my face sticky?"

Cravings are tough, but there is hope. The bottom line is that when you eat a legit Paleo diet without cheating for three or four weeks (yes, that means *in a row*), you will become fat-adapted and regain your self-control and sanity. However, every time you cheat during that intro period will most likely knock you back to square one. This is why we like to say that you aren't cheating in the beginning but that you just haven't started yet. That doesn't mean you have to start by jumping to perfect Paleo immediately, but it does mean that you should eventually get there and stay there long enough to overcome your cravings and become the fat-adapted specimen of perfect human health you were meant to be. Then the occasional cheat is not a problem. In the meantime, you will just have to summon some will power, knowing all the while that your temporary trials and tribulations are just that—temporary. Once you get to the other side you will feel great, perform well, and live long in a body that's easy on the eyes because it is actually healthy.

## Healthy Carbohydrate Consumption

"How many carbs should I eat per day?" This is a question I hear almost daily. I understand how tough it can be to change your perspective when total carbs, fat, and protein is all that seems to matter to the rest of the world, but as I have already said, you did not evolve to eat macronutrients; you evolved to eat food. Most people won't need to count carbs at all. Simply cutting out processed foods usually means that you won't be able to eat an unhealthy amount of carbs. For fat loss, avoiding starchy, but otherwise Paleo-approved, carbs is also advisable. Sweet potatoes, yams, and butternut squash are perfectly fine for athletes and those without a fat-loss goal.

"Ketones," or "ketone bodies," are used for energy when glucose and glycogen stores are depleted. The state of elevated ketone bodies in the bloodstream is called "ketosis" and indicates that body fat is the primary energy source at that time. Ketosis is perfectly natural and not harmful, although it is occasionally confused with ketoacidosis, a condition sometimes seen in diabetics and severe alcoholics in which ketones in the blood reach toxic levels. Ketoacidosis is not a side effect of healthy people eating too few carbohydrates.

The Atkins Diet is based heavily on this concept and requires reducing carbohydrates to very low levels to induce ketosis and fat loss. In truth, it did work for many people, although most had trouble sustaining it. Dr. Atkins was not too far off base, in my opinion, but ketosis is an extreme state and not really necessary. In fact, if you are not fat-adapted, ketosis can sometimes be stressful enough to inhibit you from making progress. On many occasions I have seen that an increase in vegetables or a change to starchier vegetables was all it took to get someone back on track after carb intake had accidentally drifted too low and, therefore, too stressful on the body. In my experience, the best results come at a natural, maybe even seasonally cyclic, level of carbohydrate consumption based on real food: Prolonged periods of ketosis are not recommended.

In summary, carbs are not the root of all evil, but processed carbs come pretty close. And while the appropriate amount of carbohydrates will vary from individual to individual, none of this is the first order of business. The first thing that should be addressed is eating human food. From there, I recommend that you earn your carbs. If you are not exercising (Shame on you!), you should consume fewer carbohydrates. If you are working out like a beast and are concerned with performance, you will probably need more carbs, but you will have to do a little experimenting to find the amount that works best for you. It is also very important to understand that simply eating Paleo-approved carbohydrates is not enough if they are being consumed in forms and quantities that are not found in nature. Eating right does not have to be complicated, but you will need to use your head. When your perspective is right, everything will fall into place.

# CHAPTER 9

## the practice game

### What Does Paleo Look Like?

Now that you understand the basics of Paleo food choices, you are probably picturing steak and broccoli at every meal, no variety, and lots of misery. I get it. When Western staples like grains have been an integral part of your diet for as long as you can remember, other food choices might not come to mind without a little help.

Below is our Twenty-One Day Jump-Start meal plan from Everyday Paleo Lifestyle and Fitness, the online training community that I created with my partner and dear friend, Sarah Fragoso. All of these recipes are Sarah's creations and can be found at www.everydaypaleo.com. Her amazing books, *Everyday Paleo* and the *Everyday Paleo Family Cookbook*, are indispensable to every Paleo kitchen. It is by virtue of Sarah's unadulterated awesomeness that I am sharing these recipes with you here. They should give you a good idea of what twenty-one days of Paleo might look and taste like. You get recipes for three meals a day, but this is not a cookbook, so don't expect glossy pictures of my ugly mug in the kitchen—the amount of airbrushing required to make me marketable would have driven the cost of this book into the hundreds of dollars!

# *Day 1*

## Breakfast
### *Egg Cupcakes*

*10-12 eggs, whisked well*

*1 green onion*

*2 zucchini, cut into large chunks*

*1 cup roasted red and yellow peppers, drained*

*6-8 slices bacon, cooked*

*3 big handfuls spinach*

*Sea salt and freshly ground black pepper to taste*

1. Preheat the oven to 350 degrees and generously grease two muffin tins with butter or ghee.
2. Place the eggs in a large bowl and whisk.
3. Place the green onion, zucchini, peppers, and bacon in a food processor and pulse until finely chopped but not mushy.
4. Add the bacon-and-veggie mixture to the eggs.
5. Place the spinach in the food processor and finely chop, but again, be careful not to overprocess.
6. Add the spinach to the egg mixture.
7. Stir the egg mixture well, and use a ¼-cup measure to scoop the mixture into the greased muffin tins. (You'll be able to make 18 to 20 cupcakes.)
8. Bake for 20 to 25 minutes, or until the eggs are set in the middle.

These are great to take on the go and are good with sliced avocado and green salsa.

Yield: 9 to 10 servings.

# Lunch
## *Fast Shrimp*

*2 tablespoons coconut oil*

*½ medium yellow onion, diced*

*1 red bell pepper, diced*

*1 pound wild caught shrimp (or other shrimp of your choice), deveined and tails removed*

*4 cups baby spinach leaves*

*2 tablespoons full-fat canned unsweetened coconut milk*

*½ tablespoon curry powder (or more to taste)*

*Sea salt and freshly ground black pepper to taste*

1. In a large skillet, heat the coconut oil over medium heat.
2. Add the onion and pepper and cook until tender.
3. Add the shrimp and spinach and cook for 3 to 4 minutes, or until the shrimp curl up and are no longer opaque in the middle.
4. Add the coconut milk and spices, mix well, and serve!

Yield: 3 to 4 servings.

# Dinner
## *Spaghetti in Creamy Tomato Sauce*

*1 tablespoon coconut oil*

*2 pounds mild Italian sausage or grass-fed ground beef*

*½ red onion, diced*

*3 small leeks, diced*

*1 red bell pepper, sliced thin*

*1 14.5-ounce can organic diced tomatoes*

*2 tablespoons full-fat canned unsweetened coconut milk or heavy cream*

*1 clove garlic, minced*

*2 tablespoons fresh rosemary, minced*

*Sea salt and freshly ground black pepper to taste*

*1 14-ounce can artichoke hearts packed in water, drained and cut into quarters*

*5 zucchini, sliced thin like noodles (using a julienne slicer or a spiralizer is best)*

1. In a large skillet or wok heat the coconut oil.

2. Brown the sausage or ground beef in the coconut oil.

3. Add the onion, leeks, and bell pepper to the beef and cook until the veggies are tender. Remove from heat and set aside.

4. Place the diced tomatoes with their juice in a medium saucepan and stir in the coconut milk or heavy cream. Bring to a simmer, add the garlic, rosemary, and salt and pepper to taste and stir well.

5. Add the artichokes and zucchini to the meat and veggies and then the sauce.

6. Place over low heat, stir well, and cook for another 5 to 6 minutes, just until the zucchini are al dente. Do not overcook or the "noodles" will turn to mush!

Yield: 5 servings.

# Day 2

## Breakfast
### Broccoli Frittata

*2 tablespoons grass-fed butter or coconut oil*

*½ small red onion, diced*

*1½ cups finely chopped broccoli florets*

*1 cup diced mushrooms*

*10 eggs*

*1 teaspoon granulated garlic*

*Sea salt and freshly ground black pepper to taste*

1. Place the butter or coconut oil in a large pan and melt over medium heat.

2. Add the onion and sauté until it begins to turn brown and caramelize.

3. Add the broccoli and mushrooms to the pan and sauté for 4 to 5 minutes, or until the broccoli is tender.

4. Spread the veggie mixture evenly over the bottom of the pan.

5. Place the eggs in a large bowl, add the garlic and salt and pepper, and whisk.

6. Gently pour the eggs over the veggie mixture. Do not disturb the eggs; let them cook over low to medium-low heat until the edges start to firm.

7. Place the skillet in the oven under the broiler and turn the broiler to high. Watch carefully and broil until the eggs are set through and golden brown on top.

8. Remove immediately, slice like a pizza, and serve.

Yield: 5 to 6 servings.

# Lunch
## *The Kitchen Sink Salad*

**Salad**

*4 chicken breasts, cooked and diced*

*4 hard-boiled eggs, cooled, peeled, and diced*

*½ small head purple cabbage, diced*

*1 English cucumber, diced*

*1 cup finely chopped broccoli*

*¼ cup sliced almonds*

*¼ cup chopped Italian flat-leaf parsley*

**Dressing**

*3-4 tablespoons extra-virgin olive oil*

*1 tablespoon balsamic vinegar (or more to taste)*

*½ teaspoon spicy brown mustard*

*1 teaspoon dill*

*Sea salt and freshly ground black pepper to taste*

1. Place all the salad ingredients in a large bowl.
2. Place the dressing ingredients in a small bowl and whisk.
3. Pour the dressing over the salad, toss well, and enjoy!

Yield: 4 to 5 servings.

# Dinner
## *Smoky Roast with Sautéed Asparagus*

**Coffee Spice Rub**

*2 tablespoons freshly ground coffee*

*½ teaspoon chipotle powder*

*1 teaspoon unsweetened cocoa powder*

*¼ teaspoon cinnamon*

*½ tablespoon granulated garlic*

*1 tablespoon dried oregano*

*1 tablespoon cumin*

*1 teaspoon sea salt*

**Roast**

*½ tablespoon coconut oil*

*2½ pounds grass-fed beef chuck roast*

*1 large red onion, halved and sliced*

*¾ cup water*

**Asparagus**

*2 tablespoons coconut oil*

*1 bunch asparagus, trimmed and cut into bite-size pieces*

*Sea salt and freshly ground black pepper to taste*

1. Mix all the spice rub ingredients together in a small bowl and set aside.

2. To make the roast, place the coconut oil in a large skillet and heat over medium to medium-high heat. Make sure your pan is nice and hot!

3. Massage the spice rub mixture into and all over the roast—put your hands thoroughly into the job; do not just brush it on!

4. Using tongs, place the roast in the hot skillet and sear for 3 to 4 minutes on each side. If your pan is not hot enough you will lose your spices, but if it's too hot, you will burn your roast. You want the spices to form a nice crust on the meat.

5. Place the onion in the bottom of a slow cooker and pour in the water.

6. Cover and cook on high for 5 to 6 hours, or on low for 7 to 8 hours.

7. To prepare the asparagus, melt the coconut oil in a large skillet over medium heat and sauté the asparagus until crisp but tender. Season with a little bit of salt and pepper.

Yield: 5 to 6 servings.

# Day 3

## Breakfast
### Perfect Poached Eggs with Bacon

*As many slices bacon as you need to feed your family*
*As many eggs as you would like, typically 2 to 3 per person*

1. Cook the bacon and set it aside.
2. Bring a small pot of water to a rapid boil
3. Crack one egg, being careful to keep the yolk intact, and slip the egg into the boiling water.
4. With a small spoon, keep the water moving by gently sweeping the water above the egg.
5. After a minute or two use the spoon to lift the egg out of the water to check to see if it's done: the perfect poached egg will have an opaque white and a bright yellow yolk.
6. Serve immediately with bacon.

Yield: However many servings you need!

## Lunch
### Leftover Smoky Roast and Asparagus

# Dinner
## *Chicken Wraps*

**Wraps**

4-5 chicken breasts

2 cloves garlic, minced

3 tablespoons coconut aminos
or tamari (not soy sauce, which
contains gluten)

½ cup chicken broth

2 tablespoons coconut oil

2 small zucchinis, diced

6-8 mushrooms, diced

2 teaspoons sesame oil, or more

1 head iceberg lettuce, cored,
leaves removed

**Condiments**

2 cups shredded green or purple
cabbage

1 red bell pepper, finely chopped

3 green onions, chopped

1 8-ounce can water chestnuts, diced

½ cup sliced or slivered almonds

2-3 small carrots, finely chopped

Hot chili oil to taste

1. To make the wraps, place the chicken in a slow cooker and add the garlic, coconut aminos or tamari, and chicken broth. Cook on low for 4 to 6 hours, or until the meat shreds easily.

2. Melt the coconut oil in a large skillet over medium heat, add the zucchini and mushrooms, and sauté until tender.

3. Add the shredded chicken and 2 teaspoons sesame oil to the skillet and stir well.

4. To serve, place the chicken mixture in a lettuce leaf, add condiments of choice, and wrap it up.

5. If desired, drizzle the wraps with more sesame oil and hot chili oil.

Yield: 5 servings.

# Day 4

## Breakfast
## Baked Eggs

*2 tablespoons coconut oil*

*1 sweet potato, peeled and grated*

*4 green onions, diced*

*2 cups baby spinach leaves*

*½ teaspoon smoked paprika*

*Sea salt and freshly ground black pepper to taste*

*5 eggs*

*5 slices bacon, cooked and crumbled*

1. Preheat the oven to 350 degrees.
2. Heat the coconut oil in a small skillet over medium heat, add the sweet potato, and sauté for about 2 minutes.
3. Add the green onion and cook for another minute or two. Add the spinach and cook until the spinach is just wilted.
4. Add the paprika, sea salt and pepper, and mix well.
5. Divide the veggie mixture evenly among 5 ramekins.
6. Carefully crack one egg into each ramekin.
7. Place the ramekins on a baking sheet and bake for 15 minutes
8. Remove the eggs from the oven, sprinkle each with the bacon, and bake for an additional 3 to 5 minutes, or until the whites are set but the yolks are still a little bit "jiggly."
9. Remove from the oven, carefully scoop the eggs out of the ramekins, and place in bowls to serve. Be creative with your ingredients—you can rock these a million ways!

Yield: 5 servings (but most people can't eat just one, so you might want to double the recipe)!

# Lunch
## *Mango Chicken Salad with Chipotle Mayo*

*4-5 slices bacon, diced*

*½ cup red bell pepper, diced*

*1 jalapeño pepper, seeded and finely diced*

*3 cups cooked chicken, diced*

*1 cup mango, diced*

*¼ teaspoon chipotle powder, or more or less to taste*

*½ cup homemade* Paleo Mayo *(recipe at* www.everydaypaleo.com*)*

*Shredded romaine lettuce leaves*

*Sliced almonds, optional*

1. Place the bacon in a medium skillet over medium heat and cook until almost crisp.

2. Add the red pepper and jalapeño and cook until the peppers are soft and the bacon is completely crisped.

3. Add the chicken and cook until warmed through.

4. Add the mango and stir just until warmed through, about another 2 minutes.

5. Stir the chipotle powder into the mayo.

To serve, place a pile of romaine on each of 2 plates, top with a scoop of the chicken mixture, then drizzle with the chipotle mayo. Garnish with sliced almonds if desired.

Yield: 2 servings.

# Dinner
## *Everyday Paleo Pancit*

*2 tablespoons coconut oil*

*1½ pounds chicken breasts, cut into bite-size pieces*

*1 pound pork loin, cut into bite-size pieces*

*8 green onions, diced*

*2 teaspoons crushed garlic*

*6-8 cups shredded green cabbage*

*4 carrots, grated*

*½ pound shrimp, deveined and tails removed*

*¼ cup coconut aminos or tamari*

*¼ cup chicken broth*

*2 tablespoons fish sauce*

*Freshly ground black pepper to taste*

*Lemon wedges*

1. Place the coconut oil in a large wok or skillet and heat over medium to medium-high heat. When the pan is nice and hot, add the chicken, pork, green onions, and garlic, and sauté for about 6 to 7 minutes, or until the meat is cooked all the way through but still tender.

2. Remove the meat from the pan and set aside.

3. Add the cabbage and carrots to the pan and cook until the cabbage is tender, about 4 minutes.

4. Add the shrimp to the pan and sauté with the veggies until the shrimp turns pink.

5. Return the chicken and pork to the pan and add the coconut aminos or tamari, chicken broth, and fish sauce.

6. Season with lots of black pepper, stir well, and cook for another minute or two.

7. To serve, divide among 5 bowls and include a lemon wedge.

Yield: 5 servings.

# Day 5

## Breakfast
### Coconut Milk and Curry Frittata

*1 tablespoon coconut oil*

*½ red onion, finely diced*

*7 eggs*

*¼ cup full-fat canned unsweetened coconut milk*

*2 tablespoons tomato paste*

*1 tablespoon curry powder*

*Sea salt to taste*

*2 cups fresh spinach, chopped*

1. Place the coconut oil in a 10-inch ovenproof skillet over medium heat, add the onion, and cook until it begins to caramelize.

2. Meanwhile, place the eggs, coconut milk, tomato paste, curry powder, and salt in a medium bowl, whisk to combine, and set aside.

3. Add the spinach to the onion and cook until the spinach is wilted.

4. Spread the onion-and-spinach mixture evenly over the bottom of the skillet and pour in the egg mixture.

5. Cover and cook over medium-low heat for 4 minutes. Remove the lid and transfer the skillet to the oven and cook under the broiler for another 2 to 3 minutes, or until the frittata is cooked all the way through.

6. Slice like a pizza and serve.

Yield: 3 to 4 servings.

## Lunch
### Leftover Everyday Paleo Pancit

# Dinner
## *Caldo de Pollo*

*6 cups chicken broth*

*5 carrots, diced*

*1 red onion, diced*

*1 14½-ounce can diced tomatoes*

*1 cup jarred green salsa*

*1 clove garlic, minced*

*1 tablespoon cumin*

*1 tablespoon oregano*

*1 teaspoon smoked paprika*

*⅛ teaspoon cayenne pepper*

*Sea salt and freshly ground black pepper to taste*

*4 cups cooked and shredded chicken*

**Garnish**

*Diced avocado*

*Fresh chopped cilantro leaves*

1. Place the chicken broth in a large soup pot.
2. Add the remaining ingredients, except the chicken, mix well, and simmer for 25 to 30 minutes, or until the carrots are tender.
3. Add the chicken and return to a simmer.
4. Taste and add more seasoning if desired. If you like it spicier, kick up the cayenne pepper and cumin!
5. Ladle into bowls and top with diced avocado and cilantro!

Yield: 5 servings.

# *Day 6*

## Breakfast
### *Smoked Salmon Casserole*

*4½ cups small cauliflower florets*

*1 cup asparagus, finely diced*

*4 ounces smoked salmon, finely diced*

*10 eggs*

*¼ cup heavy cream or full-fat canned unsweetened coconut milk*

*⅓ cup chives, finely diced*

*1 tablespoon fresh dill, finely diced, or 2 teaspoons dry dill*

*Lots of freshly ground black pepper*

1. Preheat the oven to 350 degrees.
2. Steam the cauliflower for 4 to 6 minutes, or until the florets are tender but not mushy.
3. Spread the cauliflower on the bottom of a 9-by-13-inch glass baking dish and layer the diced asparagus on top.
4. Layer the smoked salmon over the asparagus.
5. Place the eggs, cream, chives, dill, and black pepper in a medium bowl and whisk to combine.
6. Pour the egg mixture evenly over the veggies and salmon and bake in the preheated oven for 35 to 40 minutes, or cooked all the way through.
7. Cut into squares and serve.

Yield: 6 to 7 servings.

## Lunch
### *Chicken-Jicama Slaw*

*3 cups cooked chicken, diced (rotisserie chicken works well)*

*2 cups broccoli slaw or shredded green cabbage*

*½ cup cucumber, diced*

*½ small red onion, finely diced*

*1 cup diced jicama*

*½ cup Paleo Mayo (recipe at www.everydaypaleo.com)*

*1 tablespoon balsamic vinegar*

*1 teaspoon paprika*

*½ teaspoon chili powder*

*Pinch cayenne pepper*

Place all the ingredients in a large bowl, mix, and enjoy!

Yield: 4 servings.

## Dinner
### *Moroccan Burgers and Beet Salad*

**Moroccan Burgers**

*2 pounds grass-fed ground beef*

*2 tablespoons finely chopped fresh cilantro leaves*

*2 tablespoons finely chopped Italian flat-leaf parsley leaves*

*2 cloves garlic, minced*

*2 teaspoons ground cumin*

*½ teaspoon cinnamon*

*¼ teaspoon Penzeys Galena Street Rib and Chicken Rub (available at www.penzeys.com) or ½ teaspoon paprika and a pinch cayenne pepper*

*Lettuce leaves*

1.  Place all the ingredients except the lettuce leaves in a large bowl and mix well.

2.  Form into patties and grill or pan-fry over medium heat until cooked to your liking, about 4 to 5 minutes per side for a medium burger.

3.  To serve, wrap in lettuce leaves

Yield: Approximately 8 to 10 burgers.


**Moroccan Beet Salad**

*4 large beets (to yield about 3 cups diced after cooking)*

*1 tablespoon extra-virgin olive oil*

*1 tablespoon lemon juice, or more to taste*

*2 tablespoons chopped Italian flat-leaf parsley*

*¼ cup thinly sliced red onion*

*1 teaspoon ground cumin*

*Sea salt to taste*


1.  Wash the beets and cut them in half (leaving the skin on). If you have a pressure cooker, place them in the bottom of the pressure cooker, add about 2 cups of water, lock the lid, and bring to pressure over high heat. Turn heat to low and cook for 15 minutes, or until tender. If you do not have a pressure cooker, put the beets in a pot, cover with water, bring to a boil, and simmer until fork tender, about 15 to 20 minutes. Remove the beets from the pressure cooker or pot and set aside to cool.

2.  Peel the cooled beets, dice into bite-size pieces, and place in a medium mixing bowl.

3.  Add the remaining ingredients and mix well.

4.  Let chill in the fridge for 15 minutes before serving.

Yield: 6 to 8 servings.

# Day 7

## Breakfast
### Leftover Smoked Salmon Casserole

## Lunch
### Two-Minute Tuna Salad

*1 large head red-leaf lettuce (or other lettuce of your choice), torn into small pieces*

*2 big handfuls spinach*

*5 celery stalks, diced*

*4 6-ounce cans tuna, drained and crumbled (I use Wild Planet brand, which I happily found at Costco! Also feel free to use canned or fresh wild-caught salmon.)*

*4 hard-boiled eggs, diced*

*⅓ cup extra-virgin olive oil*

*3 tablespoons apple cider vinegar*

*2-3 cloves garlic, minced*

*Sea salt and freshly ground black pepper to taste*

*3 tablespoons capers*

1. Place lettuce, spinach, and celery in a large bowl.
2. Add the tuna and eggs.
3. Place the olive oil, vinegar, garlic, and salt and pepper in a small bowl and whisk to combine.
4. Drizzle the dressing over the salad, add the capers, toss, and serve!

Yield: 3 to 4 servings.

# Dinner
## *Spice-Rub Slow-Cooked Chicken*

*1 white onion, sliced*

*1 teaspoon sea salt*

*2 teaspoons paprika*

*1 teaspoon cayenne pepper*

*1 teaspoon freshly ground black pepper*

*1 teaspoon poultry seasoning*

*1 teaspoon granulated garlic*

*1 5- to 6-pound free-range organic chicken, giblets removed, rinsed, and patted dry with paper towels*

1. Place the sliced onion in the bottom of a slow cooker.
2. Place all the spices in a small bowl, mix well, then rub over the entire chicken.
3. Place the chicken in the slow cooker over the onion, cover, and cook on low for 5 to 6 hours (depending on your slow cooker). No need for any liquid—the chicken will cook in its own juices. Make sure to spoon the onion and some of the juices over the chicken when you serve it.

A nice side to this dish is Brussels sprouts, steamed for 5 minutes and then sautéed with a little coconut oil, dried dill, garlic, and pepper.

Yield: 5 to 6 servings.

# Day 8

## Breakfast
### Sausage Frittata

*3 tablespoons coconut oil*

*1 pound mild Italian sausage (Check out US Wellness Meats, www.uswellnessmeats.com, for quality sausage options)*

*1 medium sweet potato, peeled and grated*

*4 green onions, diced*

*10 eggs*

*Freshly ground black pepper to taste*

1. Place the coconut oil in a large ovenproof skillet and melt over medium heat.
2. Crumble in the sausage (remove from casing if necessary) and brown.
3. Add the sweet potato and cook until the potatoes are tender.
4. Add the green onions and sauté for another 2 to 3 minutes.
5. Spread the sausage mixture evenly over the bottom of the skillet.
6. Place the eggs in a medium bowl, whisk, and then pour evenly over the sausage mixture. Sprinkle with black pepper.
7. Cook for about 3 minutes, or until bubbly and you can see that the edges of the frittata are almost done.
8. Transfer to the top rack of the oven under the broiler and broil on low until the frittata is cooked all the way through.
9. Slice like a pizza and serve.

Yield: 3 to 4 servings.

# Lunch
## *Portobello Mushroom Sandwich*

*2 tablespoons coconut oil*

*2 giant portobello mushrooms, stems and gills (underside of the cap) removed*

*2 tablespoons Paleo Mayo (recipe at www.everydaypaleo.com)*

*1 cup cooked shredded chicken (you can use leftover Spice-Rub Chicken)*

*½ small yellow onion, thinly sliced*

*3 slices cooked bacon*

*1 cup arugula*

1. Place the coconut oil in a large skillet and melt over medium heat.
2. Add the mushrooms, cap side up, and cook on each side for about 5 minutes, until the mushrooms soften and start to turn golden on top.
3. Remove the mushrooms from the pan and slather each side with the mayo.
4. Pile the chicken, onion, bacon, and arugula on one half, put the halves together like a sandwich and dig in.

Yield: 1 to 2 servings.

# Dinner
## Paleo Tacos with Purple-Cabbage Slaw

**Purple Cabbage Slaw**

*3 cups purple cabbage, chopped*

*1 cup chopped cucumber*

*⅓ cup finely chopped purple onion*

*½ cup diced green mango*

*3 tablespoons olive oil*

*2 teaspoons balsamic vinegar*

*Sea salt and freshly ground black pepper to taste*

Place all the ingredients in a large mixing bowl and combine well.

**Tacos**

*2 pounds grass-fed ground beef*

*2 cloves garlic, minced*

*1 teaspoon freshly ground black pepper*

*1 tablespoon cumin*

*2 tablespoons chili powder*

*¼ cup salsa verde (green salsa) of your choice*

*Romaine lettuce leaves*

**Garnish**

*2 avocados, sliced*

*1 bunch cilantro, diced*

1. Place the meat in a large skillet over medium heat and brown.
2. Add the garlic, spices, and salsa, stir, and let simmer for 2 to 3 minutes.
3. Make tacos by placing some meat on a lettuce leaf topped with Purple-Cabbage Slaw, avocado, and fresh cilantro.

Yield: 5 servings.

# *Day 9*

## Breakfast
## *Sun-Dried-Tomato Scramble*

*1 tablespoon coconut oil, ghee, or butter*

*½ red onion, sliced*

*1 red bell pepper, sliced*

*6-8 stalks asparagus*

*6 eggs*

*½ cup marinated artichoke hearts*

*¼ cup sun-dried tomatoes*

1. Place the coconut oil in a medium skillet and heat over medium heat.
2. Add the onion and bell pepper and sauté until tender.
3. Add the asparagus and sauté until tender but still crisp.
4. Add the eggs and scramble together until the eggs are firm.

Yield: 2 to 3 servings.

# Lunch
## *Easy Ground Beef and Spinach*

*1 tablespoon coconut oil*

*½ red onion, diced*

*2 pounds grass-fed ground beef*

*5 cups fresh spinach leaves, chopped*

*2 cloves garlic, minced*

*½-1 tablespoon balsamic vinegar*

*Sea salt and freshly ground black pepper to taste*

1. Place the coconut oil in a large skillet over medium heat, add the onion, and sauté until translucent.
2. Add the ground beef and brown.
3. Add the spinach, garlic, balsamic vinegar, and salt and pepper, and cook for 3 to 5 minutes more, or until the spinach is wilted.

Yield: 5 to 6 servings.

# Dinner
## *Gingered Carrots with Mahi Mahi*

3 tablespoons grass-fed butter
or coconut oil

4 carrots, sliced

½ cup chicken broth

1 tablespoon coconut aminos
or ½ teaspoon tamari

Freshly ground black pepper

5 green onions, diced

1 tablespoon fresh lemon juice

½ teaspoon fresh grated ginger

1 teaspoon crushed garlic

Sea salt

1 pound mahi mahi or other white
fish of your choice

1. Place 2 tablespoons of the butter in a medium skillet over medium heat, add the carrots, and sauté for 5 to 7 minutes, or until they start to brown.

2. Meanwhile, place the chicken broth, aminos and pepper in a small bowl, whisk to combine, and set aside.

3. Add the green onions to the carrots and cook for another minute.

4. Add the lemon juice, ginger, and garlic to the skillet, and sauté just until the veggies are coated with the ginger and garlic.

5. Sprinkle with a little sea salt, stir again, then remove the mixture from the skillet and set aside.

6. Add the remaining tablespoon of butter to the skillet and melt over medium heat.

7. Add the fish pieces and cook for 1 minute on each side, making sure that your pan is nice and hot so that the fish sears and turns golden brown on each side.

8. Now pour the chicken broth mixture over the fish, cover, and cook for another minute or two, or until the fish is tender and flakes easily. Do not overcook!

9. Serve the fish over the gingered carrots.

Yield: 2 to 3 servings.

# Day 10

## Breakfast
### Breakfast Pizza

**Crust**

2 tablespoons olive oil

3 cloves garlic, minced

8 eggs

1 tablespoon basil

Pinch sea salt

Freshly ground black pepper
to taste

**Toppings**

1 pound ground mild Italian pork
sausage

½ cup marinara sauce (make sure it's
sugar- and gluten-free)

1-2 sweet bell peppers, diced

2 Roma tomatoes, sliced

1 cup sliced black olives

3 green onions, diced

1. To make the crust, place the olive oil in a large skillet over medium-high heat, add the garlic, and sauté for 2 minutes.

2. While the garlic is cooking, place the eggs in a medium bowl with the basil, sea salt, and pepper and scramble to mix well.

3. Pour the egg mixture into the skillet and turn the heat down to medium. Cover and let cook for about 3 minutes, or until the bottom of the eggs is set and firm. Do not stir or disturb the eggs while they're cooking.

4. Meanwhile, to make the toppings, place the sausage in a medium skillet over medium heat, brown, and set aside.

5. Remove the lid from the eggs, transfer the skillet to the oven, and broil for another 3 minutes, or until the top of the eggs is also firm.

6. Remove the eggs from the oven and spread the marinara sauce evenly on top.

7. Add the sausage and the rest of the toppings. Place the pizza back under the broiler for 5 more minutes. Slice and serve immediately.

Yield: 5 servings.

# Lunch
## *Kale Meatballs*

*1 pound pork or chicken Italian sausage (casings removed)*

*1 pound grass-fed ground beef*

*1 bunch kale, tough stems removed, leaves chopped finely in a food processor*

*½ red onion, finely diced*

*¼ teaspoon nutmeg*

*Freshly ground black pepper to taste*

*Coconut oil*

1. Preheat the oven to 375 degrees.
2. Place all the ingredients, except the coconut oil, in a large bowl, mix together by hand, and form into meatballs a little larger than golf balls.
3. Place the coconut oil in a large skillet over medium-low to medium heat, add the meatballs, and fry until browned on all sides.
4. Transfer the meatballs to a glass baking dish, cover tightly with aluminum foil, and bake in the oven for 20 minutes.

Yield: 5 to 6 servings.

# Dinner
## *Easy Skillet Rosemary Chicken*

*2 tablespoons coconut oil*

*2 pounds chicken breasts and/or thighs with skin*

*Sea salt and freshly ground black pepper to taste*

*5-6 cloves garlic, smashed and minced*

*1 yellow onion, halved and sliced*

*4 rosemary sprigs*

*Juice from ½ a lemon*

*½ cup chicken broth*

1. Place the coconut oil in a large skillet over medium-high heat. Make sure the oil is nice and hot!

2. Season both sides of the chicken pieces with the salt and pepper. Place the chicken in the hot skillet skin-side down and sear for 5 minutes, or until the skin is golden brown.

3. Use tongs to turn the chicken over, and sprinkle the garlic, onion, and rosemary on top.

4. Squeeze in the lemon and pour in the chicken broth, cover, and turn the heat down to medium-low.

5. Cook for another 15-20 minutes or until the chicken is tender.

Serve with a big green salad and olive oil and lemon juice for dressing.

Yield: 5 servings.

# Day 11

## Breakfast
### *Leftover Breakfast Pizza*

## Lunch
### *Easy Chicken Stir-Fry*

2 tablespoons bacon grease
or coconut oil

1 red onion, sliced

1½ pounds boneless, skinless chicken
breast, diced into bite-size pieces

4-5 cloves garlic, minced

Juice from ½ a lemon

¼ cup chicken broth

1 cup sliced mushrooms

1 bunch rainbow chard, chopped

½ cup diced basil leaves, fresh

1 8½-ounce can artichoke hearts,
chopped

Freshly ground black pepper to taste
(the more the better in this recipe!)

Olive oil

Sea salt to taste

1. Place the bacon grease in a large skillet over medium heat, add the onion, and sauté until it starts to brown.

2. Add the chicken and cook over medium-high heat for 3 minutes, stirring occasionally.

3. Add the garlic and cook for another minute.

4. Add the lemon juice, chicken broth, and mushrooms. Mix well and bring to a boil.

5. Cover and cook for 3 to 5 minutes more.

6. Add the chard and basil and cook until the chard is wilted, about 2 minutes.

7. Add the artichoke hearts and stir just until warm.

8. Serve with a drizzle of olive oil and a sprinkle of sea salt if desired.

Yield: 3 to 4 servings.

# Dinner
## *Paleo Enchiladas*

*2 tablespoons coconut oil, grass-fed butter, or ghee*

*1 medium onion, minced*

*2 cups tomato purée (make your own by puréeing 4 large tomatoes in a food processor)*

*4 cloves garlic, minced*

*2 tablespoons chili powder*

*½ teaspoon cumin*

*½ teaspoon oregano*

*½ teaspoon sea salt*

*1 pound seafood of choice, such as wild-caught cod, shrimp, or crab (or other protein, like shredded chicken or grass-fed ground beef. If you use chicken or ground beef, make sure that it's cooked before Step 5.)*

1. Preheat the oven to 375 degrees.

2. Place the coconut oil in a medium skillet over medium heat, add the onion, and sauté until tender.

3. Add the tomato purée, garlic, chili powder, cumin, oregano, and salt. Mix well and simmer for 20 minutes, stirring often.

4. Pour the sauce into a food processor and purée.

5. Place the seafood or other meat of your choice in a 9-by-13-inch baking dish. Pour the enchilada sauce over the seafood, cover tightly with aluminum foil, and bake in the oven for 10 to 12 minutes, or until the seafood is cooked through.

6. Serve with sliced avocados, lime wedges, and cilantro.

Yield: 2 to 3 servings.

# Day 12

## Breakfast
### *Italian Eggs*

*Cooking oil of your choice (I used bacon grease)*

*1 small yellow onion, halved and sliced*

*2-3 small zucchinis, halved and sliced*

*4-5 large tomatoes, diced*

*3 cloves garlic, minced*

*A big handful fresh basil, chopped*

*Sea salt and freshly ground black pepper to taste*

*12 eggs (more or less, depending on how big your skillet is or how many people you are feeding)*

*½ cup fresh chives, finely chopped*

1. Place the oil in a large skillet over medium heat, add the onion, and sauté until translucent.

2. Add the zucchini, tomatoes, and garlic and bring to a simmer.

3. Keep simmering the mixture, stirring occasionally until it begins to thicken.

4. Add the basil, and a little salt and pepper, stir, and adjust seasoning if necessary.

5. Make little holes in the sauce with a spoon and crack an egg into each hole.

6. Sprinkle with chives, turn the heat down to low or medium-low, cover, and let the eggs cook until the whites are done but the yolks are still runny, about 5 to 8 minutes, depending on how much sauce or how many eggs you cram into the skillet. Cook longer if you want your eggs cooked all the way through.

7. Scoop out an egg or two for each person, and enjoy!

Yield: 6 or more servings.

# Lunch
## *Ginger Beef with Mango Salsa*

**Marinade**

*¼ cup coconut aminos or tamari*

*1 tablespoon fish sauce (I recommend Red Boat Fish Sauce or Thai Kitchen)*

*1 teaspoon freshly grated ginger*

*Big pinch cayenne pepper*

*Freshly ground black pepper to taste*

**Meat**

*2 1-pound grass-fed skirt steaks*

*Lettuce leaves*

**Mango Salsa**

*1 cup finely diced mango*

*½ small red onion, thinly sliced*

*1 avocado, finely diced*

*⅓ cup finely diced cilantro leaves*

*½ teaspoon freshly grated ginger*

*1 teaspoon garlic powder*

*1 tablespoon freshly squeezed lime juice*

*2 tablespoons olive oil*

1. Heat your grill to medium-high heat.

2. Place all the marinade ingredients in a medium bowl and whisk to combine.

3. Cut each steak into 3 even pieces, add to the marinade and toss until the meat is well coated.

4. Let the meat marinate at room temperature for 20 minutes and then grill for 1 to 2 minutes on each side.

5. Remove the meat from the grill and let it rest for 10 minutes or until you are done preparing the salsa.

6. Place all the salsa ingredients in a medium bowl, toss together gently, and set aside.

7. Slice the grilled steak into thin strips.

8. To serve, place a few lettuce leaves on each plate, top with strips of steak, and finish with a large scoop of the salsa.

Yield: 5 to 6 servings.

# Dinner
## *Chicken-Chili Soup*

*2 tablespoons coconut oil or butter*

*1 small yellow onion, diced*

*4 cloves garlic, minced*

*1 jalapeño or Fresno pepper, seeds removed and finely diced*

*2 4-ounce cans diced green chilies*

*2 teaspoons cumin*

*1 tablespoon oregano*

*¼ teaspoon cayenne pepper*

*Freshly ground black pepper to taste*

*4 cups chicken broth*

*3 cups chicken breast, cooked and chopped (I used leftover grilled chicken breast)*

**Garnish**

*Chopped fresh cilantro*

*Diced avocado*

1. Place the oil in a large soup pot over medium heat, add the onion, garlic, and jalapeño, and sauté until the onion is tender.

2. Add the green chilies, cumin, oregano, cayenne pepper, and black pepper. Stir and pour in the chicken broth.

3. Bring to a boil, turn heat down to medium-low, and simmer for 10 minutes. Add the chicken and cook for 5 more minutes.

4. Ladle into bowls and garnish with fresh cilantro and avocado.

Yield: 3 to 4 servings.

# Day 13

## Breakfast
### Egg Cupcakes with Sliced Avocados
See recipe on Day 1 (page 109)

## Lunch
### Leftover Chicken-Chili Soup

## Dinner
### Everyday Paleo Salisbury Steak with Steamed Broccoli

**Steak**

2 pounds grass-fed ground beef

1 cup spinach, finely diced

1 egg

1 teaspoon crushed garlic

1 teaspoon sea salt

1 tablespoon thyme

½ teaspoon rubbed sage

¼ teaspoon marjoram

¼ teaspoon finely ground black pepper

2 tablespoons or more grass-fed butter, ghee, or coconut oil

**Gravy**

4 tablespoons grass-fed butter or ghee

1 red onion, thinly sliced

½ red bell pepper, thinly sliced

2 cups sliced mushrooms

1 cup beef broth

¼ cup full-fat canned unsweetened coconut milk

Freshly ground black pepper to taste

**Garnish**

Diced Italian flat-leaf parsley

1. Place all the ingredients for the steaks, except the butter, in a large bowl and use your hands to mix well.

2. Place the butter in a large skillet over medium-high heat. While the butter is melting, form the meat mixture into ¼-inch-thick oval patties, about 7 or 8.

3. Place the patties in the skillet, making sure to get a sizzle—the pan needs to be nice and hot!

4. Cook for 2 minutes on each side to brown evenly. You'll have to cook these in batches, so add more butter if necessary.

5. Once all the steaks are done, place in the oven to keep warm while you make the gravy.

6. In the same pan you just cooked your steaks in, melt the butter over medium heat.

7. Add the onion, bell pepper, and mushrooms and sauté until tender, about 7 to 8 minutes.

8. Add the broth and deglaze the pan (using a whisk, scrape all the bits off the bottom that remain from cooking the steaks).

9. Bring to a simmer, add the coconut milk and pepper, whisk well, and return to a simmer.

10. Turn the heat down until the gravy is just *gently* simmering.

11. Reduce the gravy by stirring frequently for about 10 minutes, until the sauce starts to thicken.

12. Once the sauce has reached desired thickness, plate the steaks, ladle some gravy over the top, and garnish with diced flat-leaf Italian parsley.

Yield: 5 servings.

# Day 14

## Breakfast
## Bacon Frittata

*2 tablespoons bacon grease, coconut oil, or grass-fed butter*

*1 8-ounce container sliced mushrooms*

*6 ounces fresh spinach*

*8 slices cooked bacon, diced*

*1 dozen eggs*

1. Place the bacon grease in a large ovenproof skillet over medium heat, add the mushrooms and spinach, and sauté until the spinach starts so wilt.

2. Add the bacon and stir.

3. Spread the bacon and veggies evenly over the bottom of the skillet.

4. Place the eggs in a medium bowl, scramble them, and pour into the skillet.

5. Turn the heat down to low, cover, and cook for about 3 to 4 minutes.

6. Remove the lid and finish the frittata in the oven under the broiler until the eggs become firm.

7. Slice like a pizza and serve.

Yield: 5 to 6 servings.

# Lunch
## *Tuna-Stuffed Eggs*

*6 hard-boiled eggs*

*2 tablespoons Paleo Mayo (recipe at www.everydaypaleo.com)*

*1 green onion, diced*

*2 teaspoons fresh lemon juice*

*2 teaspoons Dijon or yellow mustard*

*Sea salt and freshly ground black pepper to taste*

*1 5-ounce can tuna*

*Chopped pickles (optional)*

1. Peel the eggs and slice them in half lengthwise.
2. Remove the yolks and put them in a small bowl.
3. Add the mayo, green onion, lemon juice, mustard, and salt and pepper to the yolks. Mix well.
4. Stir in the tuna and mix well.
5. Spoon the tuna mixture into the hollowed-out egg halves and enjoy.

Yield: 4 servings.

# Dinner
## *Cabbage Rolls*

### Sauce

1 14.5-ounce can diced tomatoes, drained

1 cup chicken broth

1 tablespoon basil

Freshly ground black pepper to taste

### Filling

12-15 cabbage leaves

1 pound grass-fed ground beef

2 cups diced fresh spinach

1 small apple, finely diced

½ red onion, finely diced

4 cloves garlic, minced

2 tablespoons Italian flat-leaf parsley, finely chopped

1 egg

1 teaspoon paprika

1 teaspoon sea salt

1 teaspoon freshly ground black pepper

1. Place the sauce ingredients in a small bowl, mix to combine, and set aside.

2. Place the cabbage leaves in a pressure cooker with one cup of water.

3. Bring the pressure cooker up to pressure and cook for 30 seconds. Remove the leaves and set aside to cool.

4. Place the rest of the filling ingredients in a large bowl and combine well.

5. Depending on the size of your cabbage leaves, place approximately ¼ cup of filling on the bottom edge of each leaf.

6. Fold in the two outside edges of the leaf and roll up.

7. Place each cabbage roll seam side down in your pressure cooker.

8. Cover the rolls with the sauce.

9. Bring the pressure cooker up to pressure and cook for 12 minutes. Serve immediately.

Yield: 2 to 3 servings.

# *Day 15*

## Breakfast
### *Eggs fried in butter, bacon grease, or coconut oil with sautéed asparagus and chicken or pork breakfast sausage*
This one is self-explanatory

## Lunch
### *Lettuce Wraps with Thai "No Peanut" Sauce*

**Thai "No Peanut" Sauce**

*½ cup almond butter*

*½ cup full-fat canned unsweetened coconut milk or coconut cream concentrate*

*½ cup unsweetened applesauce*

*Juice from ½ a lime*

*½ tablespoon fish sauce (Red Boat Fish Sauce is great)*

*1½ teaspoons fresh grated ginger*

*½ teaspoon crushed garlic*

*Hot chili oil to taste*

Place all the ingredients in a medium mixing bowl, whisk to combine, and set aside.

**Wraps**

*2 pounds grass-fed ground beef*

*Sea salt and freshly ground black pepper to taste*

*Romaine lettuce leaves*

**Garnish**

*Chopped fresh cilantro*

*Shredded cabbage*

*Lime wedges*

1. Place the ground beef in a large skillet over medium heat, season with salt and pepper to taste, and brown.
2. Scoop the ground beef into the lettuce leaves, top with the sauce, and serve!
3. Garnish with cilantro, shredded cabbage, and lime wedges if desired.

Yield: 5 servings.

# Dinner
## *Stuffed Zucchini*

*3-4 large zucchinis*

*Extra-virgin olive oil*

*2 pounds ground bison or other ground meat*

*1 red onion, diced*

*1 eggplant, peeled and diced*

*1 8½-ounce jar sun-dried tomatoes packed in olive oil, finely chopped*

*1 cup chopped fresh basil*

*2 tablespoons finely chopped fresh rosemary*

*4 cloves garlic, minced*

*1 tablespoon oregano,*

*Splash of balsamic vinegar*

*Sea salt and freshly ground black pepper to taste*

1. Preheat the oven to 375 degrees.
2. Cut a thin lengthwise slice off each zucchini and scoop the flesh out, leaving a shell. Chop the flesh and set aside.
3. Place the shells on a baking sheet, drizzle with olive oil, and bake for 20 minutes.
4. Meanwhile, place the meat in a large skillet over medium heat to brown. When it is almost brown, add the onion, eggplant, and zucchini flesh, and cook until the eggplant is soft, about 5 to 7 minutes.
5. Add the remaining ingredients and cook for 5 to 10 minutes more.
6. Remove the shells from the oven and stuff them all as full as possible with the meat mixture.
7. Put the stuffed zucchinis back in the oven and bake for 30 to 40 more minutes.

Yield: 6 servings.

# Day 16

## Breakfast
### *Broccoli Frittata*
See Day 2 for recipe (page 112)

## Lunch
### *Chicken and Chard*

*2 tablespoons coconut oil*

*½ red onion, diced*

*1½ pounds boneless, skinless chicken breasts, cut into bite-size pieces*

*5 cloves garlic, minced*

*1 4-ounce can roasted diced green chilies*

*1 teaspoon cumin*

*⅛ teaspoon allspice*

*Sea salt and freshly ground black pepper to taste*

*2 bunches rainbow chard, roughly chopped*

*Small handful raisins and raw, sliced almonds for garnish*

1. Place the oil in a large wok or skillet and heat over medium heat.
2. Add the onion and sauté until it starts to turn translucent.
3. Add the chicken and cook for 3 to 5 minutes, or until almost cooked through.
4. Add the garlic and sauté for 2 to 3 more minutes.
5. Add the chilies, cumin, allspice, salt and pepper, and mix well.
6. Add the chard and cook until the chard is wilted, about 3 to 4 more minutes.
7. Serve with a sprinkle of raisins and almonds.

Yield: 4 servings.

## Dinner
## *Dad's Pork Chops and Sautéed Spinach*

*4 pork chops, ¼-inch thick*

*Sea salt and freshly ground black pepper, to taste*

*½ cup Dijon mustard*

*1 teaspoon mustard powder*

*1 teaspoon French thyme*

*1 teaspoon crushed garlic*

*1 tablespoon coconut oil*

1. Preheat the oven to 425 degrees.
2. Season pork chops lightly with salt and pepper.
3. In a small bowl, combine the mustard, mustard powder, thyme, and garlic; mix well and spread evenly over both sides of the chops.
4. Place the oil in a large skillet over medium-high. Add the chops and brown for 2 minutes per side.
5. Transfer the skillet to the oven and cook for 5 to 8 minutes more, until the meat is no longer pink.
6. Serve over sautéed baby spinach.

Yield: 4 servings.

# *Day 17*

## Breakfast
### *Leftover pork chops or chicken and chard*

## Lunch
### *The Kitchen Sink Salad*
See Day 2 for recipe (page 113)

## Dinner
### *Chili Colorado*

*7 dried New Mexico chilies (I recommend El Guapo brand for all the dried chilies, found at most major grocery stores.)*

*3 dried California chilies*

*3 dried Chile de Arbol*

*1 yellow onion*

*5 cloves garlic*

*2 tablespoons coconut oil*

*2½ pounds grass-fed beef stew meat*

*2 cups beef broth*

*2 6-ounce cans tomato paste*

*2 tablespoons cumin*

*2 tablespoons oregano*

*Sea salt and freshly ground black pepper to taste*

### Garnish
*Diced avocado*

*Chopped fresh cilantro*

1.  Rinse the chilies and place them in a pot with 4 cups of water.

2.  Bring to a boil, turn the heat off, and let the chilies soak in the water for 30 minutes.

3.  Meanwhile, dice the onion and mince the garlic. Place the oil in a large soup pot over medium heat and add the onion.

4.  Cook the onion until it starts to brown. Add the garlic and the beef and brown the beef, about 7 to 10 minutes.

5.  Add the broth, tomato paste, cumin, oregano, and salt and pepper to the pot.

6.  Bring to a boil, then lower heat to medium-low or low and let simmer. While the beef is simmering, it's time to prepare the peppers.

7.  Drain the peppers, reserving the soaking liquid. Remove the stems from the peppers and place the peppers in a food processor with half of the soaking liquid.

8.  Pulse the peppers until smooth. Pour the puréed peppers through a sieve into the chili pot. Use a spoon to get every bit possible through the sieve, leaving behind the seeds and any bits of pepper skin.

9.  Pour the remaining soaking liquid through the sieve into the pot. Bring to a boil, turn heat down to low, and let the chili simmer for 2 hours, or until the meat is tender.

10. Serve with diced avocado and cilantro.

Yield: 6 servings.

# Day 18

## Breakfast
### Scrambled Eggs with Leftover Chili Colorado

## Lunch
### Picnic Chicken Salad and Sliced Cucumbers

*3-4 cooked chicken breasts, diced into bite-size pieces*

*1 apple, diced*

*4 celery stalks, diced*

*1 8-ounce can sliced water chestnuts, diced*

*1 cup diced green cabbage*

*Paleo Mayo to taste (recipe at www.everydaypaleo.com)*

*Freshly ground black pepper to taste*

*1 large cucumber, sliced*

Place all the ingredients, except the sliced cucumbers, in a medium bowl and mix well. Scoop the salad up with the cucumber slices—and don't forget the napkins!

Yield: 3 to 4 servings.

# Dinner
## Ginger-Beef Stir-Fry

*2 pounds thinly sliced grass-fed flank steak or other steak of your choice*

| **Marinade** | **Veggies** |
|---|---|
| *2 teaspoons crushed garlic* | *1 purple onion, thinly sliced* |
| *¼ cup coconut aminos or tamari* | *5 carrots, julienned* |
| *2 tablespoons sesame oil, plus more for garnish* | *½ pound mushrooms, sliced* |
| *½ teaspoon freshly grated ginger* | *1 bunch baby bok choy* |
| *1 teaspoon finely ground black pepper* | |
| *Juice from 1 orange* | |

*2 tablespoons coconut oil*

1. Place the beef and the marinade ingredients in a large bowl and mix, coating the beef well. Set aside to marinate for at least one hour, but overnight in the fridge will give the meat the most flavor.
2. Place the oil in a wok or large skillet over medium heat.
3. Add the onion and sauté until it starts to become tender.
4. Add the carrots and sauté for 3 more minutes.
5. Add the beef and the marinade and sauté for 4 to 5 minutes or until the meat is cooked through but still tender.
6. Add the mushrooms and bok choy and sauté until the bok choy is wilted.
7. Serve with a few more splashes of sesame oil.

Yield: 4 to 5 servings.

# Day 19

## Breakfast
### Baked Eggs
See Day 4 for recipe (page 117)

## Lunch
### Easy-and-Amazing Roast Chicken and "No Potato" Salad

**Easy Roast Chicken**

*1 free-range 4- to 5-pound chicken, giblets removed*

*Sea salt*

1. Preheat the oven to 450 degrees.
2. Wash the chicken inside and out and thoroughly dry the cavity with paper towels.
3. Place the chicken in a roasting pan and generously sprinkle the chicken inside and out with sea salt.
4. Roast in the oven for about an hour; the chicken will be crispy golden brown on the outside and incredibly tender, juicy, flavorful, and delicious on the inside!

Yield: 4 to 5 servings.

**Everyday Paleo "No Potato" Salad**

*2 heads cauliflower*

*1 dozen eggs, hard-boiled and diced*

*½ a medium red onion, finely diced*

*6-8 celery stalks, finely diced*

*A lot of dill pickles, diced*

*About 1½ cups Paleo Mayo (recipe at www.everydaypaleo.com) with 2 tablespoons dill and 1 teaspoon crushed garlic added*

*About 1 teaspoon prepared yellow mustard*

*Freshly ground black pepper to taste*

1. Cut the cauliflower into large florets. I recommend using a pressure cooker to cook the cauliflower: place the florets in the cooker, fill the cooker with about 4 inches of water, lock the lid, bring to pressure and cook for about 2½ minutes. Remove from heat immediately and run the cooker under cold water to quickly bring down the pressure. Remove the lid and pour the cauliflower into a strainer and rinse with cold water to stop the cooking process. You want the cauliflower to be soft but not mushy! If you do not have a pressure cooker, steam the cauliflower for about 7 to 10 minutes, cooking until tender but not mushy, then place in a strainer and rinse under cold water to stop the cooking process.

2. Drain the cauliflower well and pat dry with paper towels.

3. Crumble the cauliflower into a large mixing bowl, add all of the remaining ingredients, and mix well.

4. Either eat right away or let chill for a couple of hours before serving.

This salad is HUGE and could serve at least 15 people so cut the ingredients in half unless you are feeding a crowd or want a lot of leftovers.

## Dinner
### Dry-Rub Steak with Avocado Salsa and Chopped Broccoli Salad

**Dry Rub**

¼ cup smoked paprika

3 tablespoons cumin

¼ cup chili powder

2 tablespoons Mexican oregano

1 teaspoon freshly ground black pepper

Sea salt to taste

1 steak per person, rib-eye, top sirloin, or tri-tip

Olive oil for brushing on steaks

1. Place the first 6 ingredients in a large bowl and mix.

2. Place each steak in the dry rub mixture, making sure that each side is well coated, rubbing the dry rub into the meat.

3. Let the steaks sit for at least 30 minutes at room temperature.

4. Coat each side of the steaks with a bit of olive oil before the steaks hit the grill.

I recommend top sirloin but this dry rub is great on rib eyes and flank steak too!

## Avocado Salsa

*4 avocados, diced*

*3 Roma tomatoes, diced*

*½ small red onion, minced*

*2 tablespoons fresh lemon juice*

*Sea salt and freshly ground black pepper to taste*

Place all the ingredients in a medium bowl, mix, and serve on top of your steaks!

## Chopped Broccoli Salad

*3 cups broccoli, finely chopped*

*1½ cups carrots, diced*

*1 apple, diced*

*9 slices bacon, cooked and diced*

*3 green onions, diced*

*3 tablespoons olive oil*

*2 tablespoons balsamic vinegar*

*1 tablespoon spicy brown mustard*

*1 tablespoon chopped fresh dill*

*Sea salt and freshly ground black pepper to taste*

Place all the ingredients in a medium bowl, mix, and serve!

Yield: 5 to 6 servings.

# Day 20

## Breakfast
### Leftover Steak and Avocado Salsa

## Lunch
### Leftover "No Potato" Salad and Chicken

## Dinner
### Curried Meatballs

**Meatballs**

| | |
|---|---|
| 3 pounds grass-fed ground beef | 2 tablespoons curry powder |
| 1 cup finely diced red onion | ½ tablespoon sea salt |
| 1 cup finely diced apple | Fresh ground black pepper to taste |
| 1 egg | |

1. Preheat the oven to 400 degrees.
2. Place all the meatball ingredients in a large bowl and mix well.
3. Using your hands, form the mixture into meatballs just a little bit bigger than a golf ball and place in a large, glass baking dish.
4. Bake for 25 minutes.
5. While the meatballs are cooking prepare the sauce!

**Curry Sauce**

2 tablespoons coconut oil

1 teaspoon crushed garlic

1 tablespoon raw organic honey (optional)

1 tablespoon curry powder

2 tablespoons tomato paste

½ cup chicken broth

1. Place the coconut oil in a large skillet over medium heat, add the garlic, and sauté for 2 to 3 minutes.

2. Add the honey, curry powder, and tomato paste and whisk together.

3. Add the broth and continue to whisk until the sauce is smooth. Bring to a simmer.

4. After the meatballs come out of the oven, add them to the sauce in the skillet and coat well.

5. Cover and cook for an additional 5 to 10 minutes.

Yield: 6 to 7 servings.

# Day 21

## Breakfast
## Coconut Milk and Curry Frittata
See Day 5 for recipe (page 120)

## Lunch
## Leftover Curried Meatballs

## Dinner
## Crab Cakes

*1 pound crabmeat (Chicken of the Sea "fresh" canned crab. Yes, fresh is best, but canned works just fine for crab cakes!)*

*2 tablespoons finely diced red onion*

*2 tablespoons Paleo Mayo (recipe at www.everydaypaleo.com)*

*1 teaspoon crushed garlic*

*Sea salt and freshly ground black pepper to taste*

*⅛ teaspoon chipotle powder*

*1 egg*

*2 tablespoons coconut flour (or enough to make the mixture stick together)*

*2-4 tablespoons coconut oil*

*Shredded green cabbage for serving*

*Lemon wedges for garnish*

1. If using the canned crabmeat, make sure to crumble the crab with your hands into a large mixing bowl and pick out any shells you might find.

2. Mix the crab with the onion, mayo, garlic, salt and pepper, chipotle powder, egg, and coconut flour.

3. Heat the coconut oil in a large skillet over medium heat for 1 minute, or until hot enough that a sprinkle of water in the pan makes the oil sizzle.

4. Form the crab cake mixture into palm-size patties and fry for 2 to 3 minutes on each side, or until they are golden brown.

5. Makes approximately 10 crab cakes.

6. Serve on top of the cabbage with lemon wedges.

Yield: 4 to 5 servings.

– – – – – – – – – – – – – – – – – – – – – – – – – – – – – – – – – – – – – – –

When you first saw the list of foods you would be giving up with Paleo you probably thought, "What am I supposed to eat?" But now that you have seen what twenty-one days can look like, hopefully your eyes are open to the possibilities. Let's be honest: Most of us do not eat anywhere near this much variety when left to our own devices. Sure, there were a few repeats and a few leftover meals, but there were still forty-nine unique recipes in twenty-one days. Again, this is not a cookbook, although I have tried to create a facsimile of one here. Don't let my brevity fool you—there are literally thousands of Paleo recipes to be had. If you get bored eating this way, you are not trying very hard to avoid your boredom.

# CHAPTER 10

## strong opening plays

### In the Beginning

So what now? You know which foods to avoid, which foods to enjoy, and which foods are "maybes." You have a basic understanding of the macronutrients and how they relate to Paleo. You have a little better understanding of how we store the majority of our fat and where cravings come from. You have even seen what twenty-one days of Paleo eating might look like. But it's not enough.

You may be struggling with taking the first step, despite the fact that you know you want to, because the job at hand seems too overwhelming. I have been there. It's like walking into your garage with the intention of finally getting it organized only to end up standing there dumbfounded with no clue where to begin. It feels as if nothing is where it should be and everything needs to be moved or tossed. All you want to do is go back into the house and try again another day.

Because the point is to heal your body and return to peak health, your goal needs to be at least three solid weeks of perfect Paleo with no diversions from the plan. During this time, even the "maybe" foods have to go. When you are done, you will be well on your way to a healthy gut, and you will have regained some metabolic flexibility, which will allow you to use your stored body fat for energy. This extended period of compliance is absolutely essential, but you can ease into a comfortable pace.

### The Slow Start

It's OK if you are not a rip-the-bandage-off-quickly type of person. You do not have to make every change on the same day. We have all heard the famous Lao Tzu quote, "The journey of a thousand miles begins with one step." I think in this case we could add to that quote by saying, "Any step will do, as long as it is in the general direction of your destination." Here are a few ideas to get you going with baby steps.

***Plan and eat one whole day of Paleo meals.*** Maybe you need to see that you can actually do it. If this idea appeals to you, I recommend that you try to choose an average day in your life. If your first full day of Paleo is an uneventful weekend day, you will still be left wondering if you can do it during the hustle and bustle of your busy days. Plan ahead so your nutrition will stay on course even if you end up having an extra-crazy day. Once you have one day in the bag, start planning on two days in a row. Then three. Then a week. Then...

***Start with one meal at a time.*** For example, you might set a goal to just eat Paleo dinners for your first week or two. Find a few recipes you like and make a plan for each day so there are no surprises to throw you off-course. When you have conquered one meal a day, add another, until all your meals are Paleo.

***Tackle one offensive food at a time.*** Choosing to remove grains or sugar first will return the best results because you will feel better when they're gone. Feeling better is an excellent motivator! Take a moment to plan Paleo replacements for what you're giving up. For example, if you are trying to remove grains from your diet and you normally eat sandwiches for lunch, you might choose a few Paleo lunch recipes from the 21 Day Jump-Start menu, and then plan to cook extra dinner whenever possible so you can take leftovers for lunch the next day.

***Deal with your biggest vice first.*** Sometimes when faced with the task of getting to strict Paleo there can be one particular food or drink that is nearly a deal breaker. I see this a lot with men and their beer after a hard day's work. If you have a challenging vice, you may want to start there. Making that one major change can give you the confidence to blow through the smaller changes as if they were never an issue. However, I advise you to plan a distraction. A change of routine can be a huge help. Sticking to my beer example, if you normally grab a cold one and head for the couch to watch the news, heading to the couch to watch the news without a cold one will be a lot tougher than not heading to the couch at all. You will probably be a little antsy anyway, so why not use your angst to go for a short walk? Whatever you do, make a plan before the time comes.

***Deal with your biggest vice last.*** I like this idea less than the last one, but it can work. Getting everything else right first may make your biggest obstacle seem smaller. You will be able to tell yourself, "All I have to do is give up _____ and my diet will be totally dialed in!"

Where you begin is not really crucial, as long as you begin. Whichever method you choose, take that first step with vigor and purpose, and you will soon find yourself empowered to make any and all necessary changes. Remember, the ultimate goal is to get to at least three weeks of strict Paleo. If you choose to start slow, you must keep moving! Do not get hung up on any particular baby step. You do not have license to stall your progress at every turn. Giving yourself a deadline for each step can be very helpful as long as it does not stress you out. You might, for example, say, "I think I need to start by removing grains and not worrying about anything else just yet, but I'm going to put grains behind me before next weekend so I can start working on the next step."

There is no need to let this stuff overwhelm you. If you are frozen at the starting line, it is perfectly fine to break the whole endeavor down to individual easy-to-manage projects. Everyone can get to perfect Paleo, but we all have different strengths and different ways of dealing with stressful situations. Do what works for you, but do *something*, and do it now.

# The Fast Start

Some of us are more aggressive in the way we handle our business and we do not drag anything out, even if it means things are more difficult or uncomfortable up front. If you *are* a rip-the-bandage-off-quickly type of person, by all means, dive right in. Make a plan, punch the clock, and go hard. I commend you on your fortitude and will not try to dissuade you. Many, many people have had success with this method, and I count myself among them. Please understand, though, that going full-throttle, not being willing to drag out the Paleo transition, or anything else, for that matter, may make for a little more difficulty or discomfort from the get-go: This is not an indication that Paleo is too hard or that you are a failure. You may simply need to reassess and make a new plan for another fast start, or back off a bit and try a slow-start option.

# What's the Plan?

You may have noticed that the word "plan" has come up repeatedly in the preceding sections. That was not because of my limited vocabulary. A well thought out plan is crucial. You are about to overhaul your eating habits, and while you will probably find that it is much easier than you may be thinking it's going to be, the first few steps can be precarious. This is not a time to fly by the seat of your pants.

When I say you need a plan, I mean you need a complete plan that leaves no room for you to make a misstep. Sit down in a quiet place, alone or with anyone who intends to embark on this journey with you, and write out a menu covering every meal from now until your next opportunity to write out another menu. In other words, don't plan your meals for one week if you won't have time for planning again for two weeks. Don't get too extravagant—just choose easy recipes that appeal to your palate. When you know you are in control, there will be plenty of time for pulling out all the stops and whipping up the most amazing and complicated dishes you can find. In the beginning, cravings for the junk you are abandoning can make you wish you had more time for *not* thinking about food.

Keep it simple, but be specific. If you are going for the fast start, you should know what you will be eating for lunch three days from now; otherwise you are leaving too much to chance. If your indecision about what to eat happens to coincide with someone asking you if you would like to split a pizza, you're done for. A clear and concise plan at least removes the indecision and allows you to avoid temptations that would otherwise seem like your only option. If you are in a hurry or your day suddenly spins out of control, at least your food choices will already be nailed down tight.

# *Throw It Out!*

When it comes to the practical application of Paleo nutrition, there is nothing more important then the advice I am about to give you.

*If it is not Paleo, throw it out!*

I truly believe in you, I know you can change your life in amazing ways and get yourself a brand-new body, but you probably are not strong enough to give up addicting junk food if it continues to reside within your fortress of solitude because your moments of utmost weakness will probably strike when you are relaxing at the end of your day and you have let your guard down.

Too many times I have heard, "I do so well all day, and then about an hour before bed I lose it and kill an enormous bowl of ice cream."

"You got up, put your shoes on, and drove to the store?" I ask.

"No, I got up and walked to the kitchen," s/he replies.

"Why was there ice cream in your freezer?" I ask.

"Because I ... awhile ago ... so I meant to. ... Damn, good question!"

You may succumb to Sudden Onset Weakness Syndrome for a moment or two, but a house free of temptation means this too will pass. The very second you decide to embark on your extended period of strict Paleo, you must clean out your kitchen! I don't care what you do with the contents, but it has to go.

At the risk of sounding a little harsh, you are not serious if your kitchen still harbors the enemy. Get serious.

# CHAPTER 11

## mid-game plays and game changers

### Counting Calories

The word "calorie" invokes fear in the minds of those with fat-loss goals. In fact, using the words "calorie," "saturated fat", and "cholesterol" in the same sentence is illegal in some states. OK, I may have made that up, but it is almost believable. Ask passers-by on the street how people get fat and you would probably be pounding the pavement a long time before you found someone who did not blame excess calories. That person would not be entirely wrong, but he would not be entirely right, either.

A calorie is defined as the unit of heat required to raise the temperature of one kilogram of water by one degree Celsius. In nutrition, calories are the units we use to measure the energy we get from our dietary inputs. We eat because we need energy, so just because we named these units "calories" did not suddenly mean they were on a traitorous mission to make us fat. So why do we fear calories? Our human tendency toward oversimplification is to blame.

The first law of thermodynamics says that energy cannot be created or destroyed; it can only be changed from one form to another. When applied to human physiology, it sounds like this: If more energy (calories) is consumed than is used for movement and basic bodily functions, the excess will be stored as potential energy (fat). Unfortunately, it's not quite this simple where the rubber meets the road. For example, it is easier for a highly stressed, overtrained person to store fat after eating 1,000 calories of doughnuts than it is for a healthy, fat-adapted person to store fat after eating 1,000 calories of T-bone steak. In other words, there are many other factors involved that are not taken into consideration by the first law of thermodynamics.

But calories still do technically count. If the average person increased his caloric intake by 1,000 calories per day without increasing energy expenditure, stored fat would probably increase as well. The inverse is also true. If the average person decreased his caloric intake by 1,000 calories per day, and his energy expenditure remained constant, *weight* loss would probably result. (Notice that I used the word "weight," because some valuable muscle will be lost as well as fat.) However, most of us professionals in the Paleo community have seen numerous situations in which someone actually consumed more calories after converting to Paleo yet still lost fat, sometimes in substantial quantities. It is also quite common to hear accounts of midsection fat that wouldn't budge despite severe caloric restriction. Both of these situations partly negate the "calories in calories out" theory, but it should not be ignored entirely.

Our society's obsession with trying to blame one component of our diet for our chubbiness and ill health has not paid off, and vilifying calories out of context is no exception. Having said all that, a small restriction in calories, in conjunction with solid Paleo nutrition, will usually speed fat loss as long as the total decrease is not substantial enough to cause stress to the body. As I've mentioned before, when it comes to restricting calories, a little can be a good thing while a lot can unravel your plans in a hurry and make all your progress temporary.

In a nutshell, calories count, but not enough to count them. Getting to solid Paleo by changing the types of foods you eat should be your first order of business. Then, when your body is receiving the nutrition it expects, small steps can be taken to decrease caloric intake responsibly if it seems reasonable to do so. I do not ever recommend that anyone weigh and measure food for the sole purpose of counting calories. In my opinion, calorie counting is not a psychologically healthy activity for most people, and I have yet to encounter a situation in which someone absolutely needed to know how many calories she was eating to get results. We are not research scientists administering carefully calibrated diets to subjects in a clinical trial, therefore you can give your old food scale to your stubborn friend who insists upon weighing his food in order to determine how much cardio he will need to do after work to burn it off.

My favorite way to reduce calories is to eat smaller portions at each meal and then wait about ten minutes before going for seconds. Sometimes the hormonal signals responsible for telling your brain that you have reached satiety just need a moment to catch up. If you are still hungry after a short break, go back for more, but you might find that you are comfortable and ready to leave the table. I am not recommending that you deliberately stop eating when you are clearly still hungry, only that you take a little time to listen to what your body has to say.

Reducing calories is not a tactic for the beginning of the Paleo plan, and many people never need to address calories at all. Get to solid Paleo first. There is no point worrying about how many calories you are eating if you are still eating a sandwich for lunch every day or you are drinking a bottle of wine every night. Go Paleo, and the rest will fall into place.

## *Meal Times*

When we eat is a little odd if you really think about it. First of all, breakfast, lunch, and dinner are products of industrialization. Obviously, if we must work all day, we must also plan to keep fueling ourselves. But things get weird when we start timing meals with a physiological goal in mind. Can you imagine our hunter-gatherer ancestors looking at the morning sky and exclaiming, "Oh, no! The sun is above the eastern tree line and we haven't eaten yet! We are going to get fat?" Or, "I ate too much for lunch and now I won't be able to eat an afternoon snack. If I don't eat every two hours, how will I keep my metabolism up?"

The notion that humans function best as grazers is simply not substantiated by actual human behavior. In fact, the vast majority of hunter-gatherers today eat only two meals a day, and an evening meal appears to be the most consistent and largest meal for everyone. A light meal of leftovers from the previous evening meal may be consumed in the morning before beginning the day's foray, or a light midday meal might break up the hunting and gathering, but big breakfasts and lunches are generally unheard-of.

There is value in eating more food, especially if your goal is weight gain, but if you desire fat loss, it would behoove you to return to timing your meals in a way your body understands. First of all, snacks are for kids. You do not *need* something to get you through to your next meal—your body just isn't running efficiently yet. More on that in a moment.

Second, and this one is going to blow some minds, you might consider skipping breakfast. (Great Caesar's ghost! Did he just tell me to skip the most important meal of the day?) Yes, I totally understand that you have been completely brainwashed into thinking that skipping breakfast is tantamount to cussing in church. But breakfast can be a problem, especially when we consider typical Western breakfast foods. When helping people transition to Paleo, I am regularly asked, "What will I eat for breakfast?" This question is an indication of how unnatural our *most important meal of the day* has become. Go ahead and name your ten favorite breakfast foods and then see which ones are Paleo. The list is short because we have been convinced that eating a bowlful of processed birdseed or a stack of pan-fried wheat disks smothered in high-fructose corn syrup is somehow the key to a good day. Wrong!

I am not suggesting that eating fewer times a day means eating fewer calories. I, for one, tend to eat more total calories in two meals than in three, but adding meals to my day almost instantly begins to add fat to my midsection. Many of my clients have experienced the exact same thing; others end up eating a little less in two meals than in three, but the only reason they noticed a dip in calories is that I asked them about it.

Forgoing breakfast is basically intermittent fasting without a rigid plan. Intermittent fasting is all about decreasing the window of time that food is consumed in a day, usually without restricting caloric intake. In other words, roughly the same amount of food is eaten in less time. Intermittent fasting has produced some amazing results and has shown remarkable health benefits in animals, but it can be too stressful for some people. Most of my clients have an easier time wrapping their heads around the idea of skipping breakfast and not worrying about setting a timer for the exact moment they should begin eating.

Here again we have mid-game considerations for fat loss. Don't worry about meal times and the value of breakfast if you are still working on basic Paleo. I can assure you that you will be healthier if you stop grazing, but if your food choices are still bad you have bigger fish to fry than meal counting. Once you have your Paleo ducks in a row, you will be well on your way to regaining some control over our next subject, appetite.

# Appetite

The whole point of eating fewer meals and intermittent fasting is to regain and maintain a good relationship with our friend metabolic flexibility (see page 105). To review, having good metabolic flexibility means easily switching between fat and glucose as energy sources. Paleo alone is a huge step in the right direction for most people, and many never need anything else. As discussed previously, the beginning can be a little rough, but once you are fat-adapted the cravings slip away.

There are, however, those who switch to Paleo and experience increased appetite. This tends to indicate a sort of halfway point in which adequate metabolic flexibility has not quite been reached and total calories have increased to compensate. Basically, it appears that some people reach a state in early Paleo where they are eating all the right foods and not really jonesing for their old foods, but cravings have morphed into an overall increase in consumption. In this situation, calories *do* matter and fat loss *can* stall.

If you find yourself here, step back and reassess your situation. Are you eating according to the Paleo plan? Did you go strict Paleo for a full three weeks before allowing yourself the occasional cheat? Are your cheats in fact *occasional*? If you answered yes to all of these questions, you may need to look at your total intake. If you feel hungry all the time and think that may be inhibiting your progress, try omitting breakfast, or having just two meals per day, for a week or two and see how you feel. This should not result in a large reduction in calories because your caloric intake will ideally just be consolidated in two meals rather than three.

Expect to experience a little discomfort at first. Remember, your appetite issues are most likely an indication of your not being fat-adapted yet, so in the beginning you will feel just as if you were breaking an addiction to sugar and processed carbs. Your body will be yelling "What are you doing? Eat something already!" because it has to be reminded that the pantry (your buns and thighs) is full of stored fat.

Invariably someone will read this and jump to the conclusion that starvation is the answer to fat loss. Don't be that person. We have been over this already, but remember that my recommendations to eat less often do not imply eating fewer calories. I just want to help you get your body to run as smoothly as nature intended. Since there is a good chance that you have spent your entire life eating in ways that are not conducive to what your body evolved to expect, a little change is in order. Change can be a challenge, but it is worth it when improved health is the result.

# Results May Vary

I have never seen legitimate Paleo fail to produce benefits. Even when people deviate from the plan with enough regularity to sabotage their goals, they still tend to feel better or find some modicum of relief from a disorder that they thought was just part of life. However, I have seen enormous variations along the path to success. Some people get exactly the results they want in half the time they expected by doing nothing more than basic, textbook Paleo. Others see benefits they didn't expect while their primary goal is slower to attain. It is important to remember a couple of points in order to avoid frustration.

First, you are not a machine. You are an amazing and complicated example of biology at its finest. Therefore, it is silly to expect linear results, even when results have been linear thus far. In other words, the graph of your progress will never look like a perfectly straight line from start to finish. If your waist size decreases by exactly one inch per week for six weeks and then not at all the seventh week, do not think that you are suddenly failing. There may be other amazing benefits on the way, and biochemistry is not really concerned with what we expect any stimulus to produce.

Second, the Paleo lifestyle produces results that are sustainable and last a lifetime. This is what you want. Using tricks and gimmicks to get temporary results will not leave you happy. If you are someone who responds to Paleo little more slowly than others, I understand that it can be frustrating, but take a deep breath and remember what you are trying to create. Diligence will reward you in ways that will probably exceed your own expectations. Some of the people I mention in this book made fast progress, some did not, but all will tell you it was well worth the effort.

You will be happiest if you try to look at this journey as a one-year plan. Even if you achieve remarkable results very quickly, you will still be better in a year. You will not go from normal to peak health in the blink of an eye, so settle in and enjoy the ride.

# Tweaking the Knobs and Dials

Jump ahead in time with me for a moment to a point in your journey when you have all the basics nailed down. All of the big offenders have been out of your diet for three months. You are dead serious about your fat-loss goal, so even the "maybe" foods are long gone. You eat meat at almost every meal and fill in the gaps with non-starchy vegetables. You are exercising responsibly, getting adequate sleep, and managing your stress. You are down two pant sizes and feel strong and energized. You are now comfortably Paleo, and everything has gone according to plan with excellent results up to this point, but progress is beginning to come a little slower.

You already know that progress can ebb and flow, but sometimes small adjustments along the way are called for. Please note that there is no need to even think about changing anything until at least a couple months have passed, and three or four months is an even better vantage point from which to assess your plan. Like everything else, making these adjustments requires a healthy perspective. Do not let desperation creep in and convince you to start modifying too early or too often. If your attitude has regressed a bit and you have spent some time examining your body under a magnifying glass searching for reasons to be mean to yourself, now is not the time to overhaul your game plan. When you know that you are not acting impulsively, some clear-headed experimenting can begin.

It is very important that you approach such experimentation scientifically. Changing too many variables at once is not the way to find out what works and what doesn't. For example, you might cut back your carbohydrate intake, stop eating breakfast, reduce calories a little by giving yourself more time between second helpings, and also add another day of intense conditioning exercise to each week. But what if cutting back your carbs was all you needed? What if all those other changes actually detracted from the results you could be getting from only cutting back your carbs? Even if the other changes are not detrimental, you will have no idea which tweak worked.

Along with making one change at a time, it is also important to give each change ample time to produce the results you desire. You might get good results from a specific tweak within a few weeks, maybe even a few days, but sometimes amazing benefits take longer to be realized. Don't be the person who says, "I feel like I'm not getting anywhere. I cut back on starchy carbs four days ago, and the scale still says the same thing when I weigh myself four times a day."

When it comes to experimenting, less is more. Not only is it a good idea to limit the total number of changes, but some individual changes warrant baby steps. Calories are a great example. As you already know, while a small reduction in caloric intake can be quite helpful, a large caloric restriction will probably wreck your chances for long-term success. Add or reduce calories responsibly and without desperation, or suffer the consequences.

I can't be as specific as I'd like to because everyone's situation is unique, so I am empowering you to do some detective work and find what is best for you. But please, begin tweaking the knobs and dials *after* all the big pieces are in place and have been for a while. If you follow my advice and try to leave emotion out of your experiments, you will find what works best for you.

## Extra Considerations for Fat Loss

If your primary goal is fat loss, there are a couple of things you need to know, but they may not be as important when your excess body fat is gone. Both of these subjects remain misunderstood by many people, sometimes even by those who have been living Paleo for a while. I am going to try to clear up any confusion once and for all.

### Liquid Food

Drinking calories is a bad idea if you want to lose fat. I'm sure you are already convinced of the high-badness factor of sugary soft drinks, but fruit juice and smoothies should also be avoided. Liquefying food is basically external digestion, and external digestion means that your own digestive system doesn't have to work as hard to break down what's entering your body into individual macronutrients. In the case of liquid carbohydrates, the time from ingestion to glucose in the bloodstream is shortened. If you remember the lessons in the section on carbohydrates (see page 101), more glucose in your bloodstream in less time is the opposite of what you are looking for to optimize fat loss.

I know the idea that fruit and vegetable smoothies are bad is tough to swallow because their main ingredients are all Paleo-friendly, but I have seen smoothies and juices stall fat loss in many people who immediately began making progress again when the liquid food was removed. Don't get me wrong: I love a good smoothie, but smoothies must be treated as occasional treats.

Protein shakes should not be necessary for anyone except *maybe* athletes trying to gain weight or those who are primarily concerned with strength and performance. For these select few, shakes can be used to get extra calories and protein when they can't seem to eat enough to get the job done. For example, off-season body builders often eat a very high calorie diet, and drinking some of their daily calories can be a necessity. Everyone else should be able to easily consume enough calories and protein in whole foods.

Water is the only liquid that is approved for absolutely everyone. Decaffeinated coffee and tea are fine for most people, too, but some people still experience negative effects from the small amount of caffeine left in decaf. (See page 96 for my advice on coffee and tea.) If you like a little fizz in your life, soda water (not tonic water) is probably fine occasionally, but it might not be ideal for your teeth due to acidity. If you are motivated to take up less space, ditch the liquid foods.

## Paleo Treats

When I defined Paleo for you, I told you that it is not a diet in the sense of the word that we have become accustomed to. You should not view Paleo as a set of rules to follow. Instead, you should view it from the perspective of the question "What is human food?" Unfortunately, many people never fully understand this concept. This misunderstanding is one of the top reasons that people fail when they think they are doing what they are supposed to be doing. Please make note of these very important facts:

▫ Paleo versions of non-Paleo treats are *treats* and should be treated as such. They are *not* OK for regular consumption. Eating them often *will* impede your ability to get healthy and fit.

▫ Paleo treats are not meant to be transition foods. They will not make it easier for you to switch to a Paleo lifestyle. They are not OK during your strict starting phase.

I have trained many a client who swore that he was eating exactly as he should yet still could not lose fat and was still not feeling better. After insisting that he log his food for a few days, I would find itemized quantities of modern junk preceded by the word "Paleo." "Paleo" pancakes, "Paleo" muffins, "Paleo" bread, "Paleo" cookies, "Paleo" brownies, "Paleo" cake, and even "Paleo" candy. These poor people had learned about Paleo, and believed in it, but immediately classified it as a diet. In doing so, they were convinced that they could get amazing results while eating any food that was sanctioned by the "rules" of the Paleo diet. It makes me sad to say it, but recipes for this stuff have saturated the Paleo Internet community, leading more people every day to miss the point and end up frustrated.

Although Paleo treats are technically Paleo because they use Paleo-friendly ingredients, they still usually contain processed carbohydrates in unnatural concentrations. Therefore, they are still prone to ending up on your buns and thighs. They are easier on the gut than the offenders they imitate, but they haven't lost their ability to keep you squishy, especially if they contain vast quantities of honey and maple syrup, which the creators of these recipes/products think are fine because they are natural.

Don't get me wrong: I think it's great that there is such a thing as Paleo pancakes for the rare Saturday morning that my daughters want them. It's nice to have a Paleo go-to recipe when it's your child's birthday and you want to take cupcakes to her classroom. And baking Paleo cookies can be a fun activity to share with our children. What I am dead set against is allowing anyone to believe that Paleo treats are an acceptable part of regular Paleo nutrition.

If you want topnotch results, you must completely divorce yourself from the foods that brought you to your current state, at least long enough to break free of their hold on you. Thus, Paleo treats have no place when you're a Paleo novice. Overcoming addiction is not about finding something that most closely mimics the thing you are addicted to; it is about forming new habits and moving on. Translation: Paleo treats are no better than the real thing when it comes to helping you find a healthier perspective. If you regularly *need* to eat Paleo versions of the same old foods that made you miserable, you are not yet in the healthiest place in your head. If you allow yourself to finally escape their clutch, you will not miss them. I promise.

# CHAPTER 12
## stay in the game

### Spare No Expense

One objection to eating Paleo is that it costs too much. While this is not necessarily true, and many in the Paleo community have proved that perfect Paleo is possible on a budget, I am not about to give you money-saving tips. I apologize if that is what you were hoping for. I am here to help you change the way you think, and the cost of food is a subject that reflects your mindset more than you may realize.

Let's get the potentially offensive stuff out of the way first, with the caveat that I'm not trying to be insensitive or judgmental. I understand that you may be legitimately broke. I have certainly been there myself. I only ask that you look at things for what they really are before deciding what you can and cannot afford. Everyone has his own budget, but if you truly want extraordinary health and fitness, the statement "I can't afford Paleo food," should be part of a longer statement like, "I don't have a car payment, I don't go out on the weekends, I don't go on vacations, I never eat out at restaurants, etc., and I still can't afford Paleo food." Before you torch this book and hunt me down and drag me off to the gallows, let me make it clear that I am not telling you what to prioritize; I am simply saying that putting other expenses that are not absolute necessities ahead of food is a choice. Nobody is *making* you do any of those things, just as nobody can *make* you get healthy and fit.

Now let's take a look at how you may be misunderstanding the role of food when comparing expenses. It saddens me that the huge majority of people in the Western world see purchasing food as a burden. It is very common to view grocery shopping as the one area in your life where you can scratch and claw your way to the most savings. The electric bill will go only so low, even when you turn off every light you are not using and refrain from running the air conditioner until temperatures rise into the low 150s. But the cost of groceries can be driven down by using coupons, by shopping at the right stores at the right times, and by sticking to the cheapest types of foods. The first two are fine, but the last one will kill you. And for what?

We need to back up a bit. Humans have the same basic goals as every other creature on earth: eat, breed, and try not to die. Of the three, only breeding is deemed worthy of spending without abandon. Clothing, hairstyles, tans, manicures, cosmetics, cars, jewelry, and trendy electronic gadgets? None are essential to survival but all are prized in the human mating dance. Interestingly, even in the mating dance, and even if we are only discussing physical appearance, none of those things wields a fraction of the power that proper nutrition does when it comes to making you beautiful. Nothing you can buy will disguise bad health, and as you have already learned, we are all innately attracted to displays of good health.

You are reading this because you have a desire to look better, feel better, increase your physical capacity, or some combination of the three. How do we accomplish those goals? Correct, we improve health. What do we do every single day that has an indescribably huge and unparalleled effect on our health? That's right: We eat. Are you sure the grocery store is the best place to pinch every penny regardless of sacrificing quality? These are not rhetorical questions. I am asking honestly because I can't tell you how you should answer them. I can only tell you how I would answer them, which I bet you can guess.

## Get Cooking

The unfortunate truth is that the world is not ready to cater to your Paleo needs, which means that you are going to need to become self-sufficient. Specifically, you need to know how to cook your own food. Sorry, bachelors, the selection of microwavable, processed food-like substances in the freezer at your local grocery store will no longer suffice. It is possible to eat very close to Paleo at many restaurants, but you will probably have to endure a lot of dubious vegetable oil, at the very least. Therefore, until the world catches up and Paleo-friendly food becomes more widely available outside your own kitchen, into the kitchen you must go.

But, wait, there is good news for the culinarily inept. We live in a remarkable time of free information everywhere. The Internet is ready and willing to show you how to navigate your kitchen. For example, searching YouTube for "chop vegetables" returns a slew of demonstration videos posted by nice folks who don't want you to cut off your fingers. There are even videos on how to boil water and how to use measuring cups. It's not a big deal if you need to start with the most basic basics. Just watch the videos alone and nobody will ever know.

If you are cooking only for yourself, you really need to hurry up and find only a few staple recipes and the skills necessary to not destroy them. Then you can take your time and accumulate more recipes and more skills as your tastes dictate. Cooking for the whole family may present more pressure to provide variety, and this might be a good place for an option from the Slow Start section (page 161) that would allow you to introduce Paleo foods to your family without having to learn twenty new recipes in a week.

If you already know how to cook but are not familiar with cooking Paleo-friendly, recipes abound. Sarah Fragoso's *Everyday Paleo* and *Everyday Paleo Family Cookbook*, as well as *Paleo Slow Cooking* by Chrissy Gower, are great resources to get you started, and there are thousands of recipes scattered on the Interwebs. Just be sure that liberties haven't been taken with the interpretation of what constitutes healthy Paleo foods.

I am by no means a master chef, and cooking will never be a passion of mine, so I understand completely if this part of your journey seems daunting. I just want you to understand that you will need to hold the reins if you expect to succeed. Cooking your own food may be a little less convenient than pulling your car up to a drive-through window and cramming fast food into your gullet, but it is essential. Once you know what you need to eat to get healthy and fit, don't expect anyone else to take responsibility for feeding you properly. Step up and own your new lifestyle by preparing and enjoying the foods that will carry you to peak health.

## Falling (or Jumping) Off the Wagon

I stumble sometimes. So will you. The only points worth pondering are the frequency at which you stumble and what you do when it happens.

Deviating from your plan too often eventually starts to look like not having a plan. As I have stated previously, it is essential that you begin Paleo by working toward at least three weeks of strict adherence to the basic tenets. As I already stated, little slips here and there can be considered *cheats* after rigid beginnings, whereas without a period of strict adherence, slip-ups are really just *not starting*.

It is important to note that we all live here on earth and life happens to all of us sometimes. More than once I have found myself choosing less-offensive over most-offensive because those were the only food choices available and I had decided that starvation was not an option. Looking back, I may have been a weenie and caved before it was totally necessary, but savage hunger is a strong motivator. There have also been times when I encountered junk food that had not crossed my path in a long time and I experienced momentary amnesia—forgetting how bad it had made me feel the last time I ate it. A moment is all it takes sometimes. What ensued was something like, "Yum!" followed by, "Blech!" My body wasn't the same body it had once been and knew better—thank goodness!

To return to my point, trying to keep a healthy chunk of time between your cheats is essential to your success. Fortunately, if you really go hard in the beginning and your gut has a chance to heal, cheating with most processed foods will tend to have repercussions. It may sound crazy to you if you are not already accustomed to Paleo nutrition, but what once seemed like an innocuous slice of bread can make you feel as if you ate a box of tacks.

When clarity returns after a cheat, your next move is very important. I have often heard clients plead, "I fell off the wagon and I don't know how to get back on!" My answer: "Are you actually chewing and swallowing bad food right at this very moment? No? Good—you are already back on the wagon. Keep moving forward."

We get into trouble when we cheat and then assume that one bite has ruined some ambiguous extended length of time. You know what I mean. On a random Friday morning you drink a white chocolate mocha during a momentary lapse of judgment. You instantly feel remorse and wish you could take it back, but somehow you come to the conclusion that your entire weekend is ruined, and so you cheat your way out of an entire month's worth of progress in just 3 days. To make matters worse, you have only a slim window to get things moving forward again on Monday morning or you will pronounce the whole week worthless and decide not to reset until the following Monday. Repeat this mess a couple of times and eventually it will seem as if you have been off the wagon so long that it might have left without you.

I'm going to let you in on a little secret. Are you ready? Every single second of your existence qualifies as a perfect time to get back on the wagon. If you just had a bite of something bad and regret it, make a better decision with the very next bite of food that passes your lips. If you ate an entire meal that was not on the Paleo plan, make a better decision with the very next bite of food that passes your lips. If a weekend went by while you were walking next to said wagon instead of riding in it, make a better decision with the very next bite of food that passes your lips. If it took weeks for you to regain your self-control and now you are overflowing with self-loathing and misery, make a better decision with the very next bite of food that passes your lips. Do you see a pattern here? When the question is *when*, the answer is *now*.

## Love the Process!

In my opinion, the idea of earning your cheats is a bad one. I cannot tell you how many times I have heard someone say something to the effect of, "Tuesday will finally be three weeks of strict Paleo and I can't wait to have [*insert junk food here*]!" Or, "I only cheat on Friday nights. I figure I have earned it after a whole week of strict Paleo."

As my client and friend Deb Hunter says, these people are treating Paleo as if it were a cross to bear. This attitude is an indication that they hate something about their situation, probably something about the way they look, and they are willing to endure whatever torture they must in order to escape it. In other words, they have no real desire to live this way. The Paleo lifestyle is only a means to an end. Failure lurks in the shadows.

There are also many people who want everything quantified in exact numbers. They ask questions like, "If I eat Paleo 80 percent of the time I can still get results, right?" and "How many times a week can I cheat?"

Translation: "I hate all this stuff, so just tell me exactly what I can get away with." This attitude almost always results in failure. Paleo is not a temporary trick to get temporary results. It is an overhaul of the lifestyle that turned you into the mass of frustration you are now. Getting temporary respite from that state of frustration only to return to it at a later date is madness. Paleo is intended to be permanent.

As already discussed, the people who end up being the envy of all are invariably those who love themselves enough to strive for an overall improvement in their health and vitality. They come to truly believe that their bodies deserve the best they can provide. This means that cheats aren't worth it to them. For them, the separation from the garbage foods they held so dear does not entail misery; they have let go of the emotional relationships they had with those foods that kept them from success. The way they feel now has become far too valuable for them to even consider another option.

I have always claimed that Paleo is the only way of eating that will speak for itself if given the chance. Diets are usually limited by how long you can endure being miserable. The longer you suffer, the smaller you might get before gaining all your weight back and blaming yourself. Paleo is different because everyone always feels better. Because I know where you are headed if you take this stuff seriously, I can confidently say that you will find your results to be worth much more than what you may feel you are losing at the moment. In fact, I can also confidently say that you will not even mourn the loss of what you are leaving behind. Thus, I am asking you to view these changes as a privilege and a gift to yourself. Celebrate every little step along the way. When you come to your first reward, be it a better night's sleep, or more energy in the afternoon, or better mood, or looser pants, or clearer skin, or fewer headaches, or whatever it may be, that moment of realization is deserving of a maniacal laugh and a mighty fist-pumping cheer. These results are nothing short of amazing, and inspiring, and totally worth it! When was the last time you felt that way about a bag of triple-fried tortilla chips or box of cream-filled, chocolate-glazed doughnuts?

## *You Are the Judge and Jury*

I have been told countless times that "cheat" is a negative word and should not be used to describe stumbling off the path. I disagree. If you truly want peak health and fitness, and truly have faith in the path to get you there, self-imposed obstacles *are* inherently negative in relation to your health and fitness goals, and we should call them what they are.

However, I think it's important to note that cheating is subjective. I cannot set your level of motivation for you. If I could, I would be the most successful trainer in the world, because motivation is really the deciding factor once you have discovered the Paleo path. Alas, you will decide when you have crossed the line and let yourself down. For example, there are some gray areas in Paleo, depending on your goals. If your goal is to lose excess fat as fast as possible, it might be wise to avoid starchy vegetables, so for you eating sweet potatoes might be considered a cheat.

I have trained many people who wouldn't get totally on board with their nutrition but who appeared to be happy and never complained about their health and fitness. Many of these clients have been men who ate "mostly Paleo" and experienced some nice benefits as a result, but were not willing to go the extra mile and dial it all in. They had no desire to go further, so who am I to say they aren't happy because they don't want what I want? These people are doing what makes them happy based on their goals. But make no mistake, those people, with those relaxed goals, will probably not read this book, and they are probably not you.

All of which is to say that if we can agree that cheating is subjective and based on our goals, then we can also agree that the degree to which we cheat is an accurate measure of our motivation. When motivation rises, cheating declines. In my opinion, asking me to avoid the word "cheat" is like saying, "Please don't put a negative spin on this thing that I have decided is negative." It sounds silly when I put it like that, but it's true. If you label something a *cheat*, or agree with the concept that deviating from Paleo is *cheating*, then you obviously want to reach your goals and you understand what you are doing when you step off the path. If this is clear to you, then it should make sense that your total cheats over any period of time are a much more accurate depiction of your desire to reach your goals than what you say. In other words, repeatedly saying "I want this" is irrelevant if your actions are proving otherwise.

## Make Them Ask

Paleo is exciting! The results often come quickly, you feel like a million bucks, and it is such a thrill to finally find the path you have been looking for every time you were lured in by a diet that turned out to be another trick or gimmick. Naturally you want to tell the people around you what you are doing so they can reap these same benefits and be as happy as you.

But they rip the rug out from under you, clip your wings, and break your heart by saying something like, "You're crazy! You have to eat grains! Everyone knows that!" Your whole day is ruined, and even worse, you actually find yourself questioning your choices, despite your results. As soon as you get a chance, you tell the whole miserable story to the few Paleo people you know, probably on the Internet, but these people are not the majority in your world. Tomorrow you will have to go back out there and face the doubters who think you have gone off on some wacky new tangent.

I am going to give you some powerful advice, but my publisher will probably not like it, and you may have a hard time taking it. But here we go anyway: *Stop being a Paleo evangelist!*

I know it sounds crazy coming from a Paleo professional, but this one piece of advice will save you a lot of heartache. Get on board, keep your head down, and get results. Then, when people notice what you've got and want some themselves, they will ask you what you have been up to. When you have not yet realized any results, preaching Paleo dogmatically to people who aren't curious will usually beget resistance.

I have received hundreds of emails, calls, and texts asking for information that might help people win an argument over Paleo nutrition. "Please help me!" they say. "My brother's neighbor's pool boy's aunt's banker's unicycle instructor said we need grains or else we won't be able to poop. What should I tell him?"

"Nothing," I say. "Go eat a steak."

The unicycle instructor in question is not looking to change. Trying to evangelize him will just either bring you to tears or feeling like hitting him over the head with a folding chair like a professional wrestler. Even if you could bury a huffy and indignant person in scientific answers, he probably won't see the light, at least not right then and there. People have to want answers for you to be able to offer them to them—the time has to be right.

I used to say, "Pick your battles." Now I say, "Don't do battle." Focus on your goals and change lives by example. When someone asks why you turned down the bread at a restaurant, you can usually gauge her motives by her tone. If she sounds aggressive, it probably means she's feeling judged for eating bread herself. Tell her you feel better when you don't eat bread. What can she say?

Sometimes someone will dupe you into believing he's honestly curious, only to assail you with mainstream nutrition doctrine once you say your piece. This is how to use the same strategy to escape unscathed:

Him: Why don't you eat bread? (*Honestly curious.*)

You: I'm eating Paleo now.

Him: Paleo? What's that? (*Still curious.*)

You: I don't eat any processed food, which includes grains.

Him: But grains are good for you! How can you not be eating grains? (*Now you have gone too far!*)

You: I actually feel a lot better since I quit eating grains.

Him: But where will you get your vitamins/minerals/fiber/magic unicorn dust?

You: I'll be fine. You can read up on it if you like, but I really do feel a lot better since I stopped eating grains.

Done. As before, your last statement is inarguable and ends the discussion. In this situation, you can walk away feeling fine about your choices, and the door is open for him to check out Paleo. If you had launched into an argument with him about the evils of grains, you may have caused him to feel backed into a corner, remaining stubborn so as to avoid an "I told you so" situation with you in the future. Instead, you have empowered him to investigate further while you go back to Paleo business as usual. Everybody wins!

## Can I Get Some Support Here!

Sometimes the people closest to us can become the biggest obstacles in our path despite the fact that we long for their support the most. You find what you have been looking for forever and they just roll their eyes or, worse, argue that it can't possibly work. You are heartbroken.

When you really think about it, though, you can't really blame them for their lack of support. It would be nice to have it, but these people stood by when you tried a bunch of wacky diets in the past, only to fail miserably. Your spouse or significant other, mom, dad, brother, sister, best friend, whoever may not get fired up about Paleo just because you do. You can probably remember an instance or two when someone dear to you was excited about something that seemed trivial to you. If that thing ended up reaping huge benefits for that person, you probably came around, becoming more involved and sympathetic.

For example, many couples at my gym began their journeys with one person starting months before the other. For whatever reason, and after dozens of invitations, the spouse/boyfriend/girlfriend finally submits and ends up loving it. There are also halves of couples that remained completely uninterested.

To be honest, I have never seen people succeed solely because of support from their cheerleaders. In my gym and on the forums at Everyday Paleo Lifestyle and Fitness, the communities are strong and extremely supportive. Still, the people who are driven are the ones who are successful. They find us, ask all the necessary questions, and put their noses to the grindstone. Their progress is inevitable and unstoppable. Some are talkative, sharing their progress every step of the way; some quietly stride along diligently with their heads down.

On the flip side, people have left my gym only to be convinced to return by other members, but I have never seen someone in that situation reach his goals. The members who did the convincing are all pom-poms and high kicks, but it is not enough. If your reasons for getting healthy and fit are not your own, you have a very short window of opportunity to adopt them before you begin spinning your wheels and eventually failing. In other words, it is fine to learn about the Paleo ideals from someone else, but you must fall in love with them yourself. It is your motivation, and no one else's, that counts when it comes to your success or failure.

Even when someone says, "I need to get healthy so I can be here for my kids," she is still making a conscious decision and owning it. Kids everywhere have asked their parents to take better care of themselves to no avail. Mom and/or Dad will get in shape when it becomes important enough to Mom and/or Dad.

We make changes based on our desire to reach certain goals. Nobody else eats for you. Nor do they exercise for you. Thus, their support is nice, but not essential. We do not *need* cheerleaders, and we can't blame not having them for our lack of success.

# CHAPTER 13

## eyes on the prize

### Health and Fitness by Rote

How much time do you spend worrying about taking a shower, or brushing your teeth, or getting dressed? Probably none. Most of us bathe and groom ourselves every single day and never give it a second thought. These chores are time-consuming too. Imagine what you might accomplish if you could get back all the time you have spent in your bathroom, not including visits to the toilet. Best-selling novels have been written in less time per day.

Every time you bathe, you are making a decision to do so. You do have a choice, and you are subconsciously weighing the benefits of bathing versus not bathing. You absolutely can live the rest of your life without bathing. You would not be much fun to be around, but the choice is yours. Most of us never put any thought into it, though, because we do not consider bathing an option. It is a necessity if we don't want to stink, which is a given. Therefore, we bathe by rote, usually daydreaming all the while and barely mentally present for the details.

How simple these tasks are has always struck me as odd. Nobody ever "falls off the wagon" with grooming. Nobody "cheats" on brushing his teeth. Nobody needs a support group to hold her accountable for bathing. We do certain things because they are just what must be done if we want to avoid the consequences of not doing them. Some things are simply beyond reproach. And therein lies the magic.

How are exercising and eating properly any more difficult or time-consuming than all the other daily chores we already perform without batting an eye? They are not more difficult, but for some reason the benefits of exercising and eating properly pale in comparison to the benefits of personal grooming practices. When we stop to examine the details, things get a little strange. See if you can prioritize the following statements:

I would like to avoid stinking.

I would like to avoid disease and live a long, healthy life.

Wow, that's a tough one. Both of those statements hold a lot of value for me. If I smell like the south end of a northbound donkey, my career, social life, family life, and therefore every other aspect of my life, will be negatively affected. If I develop cancer, heart disease, type 2 diabetes, or Alzheimer's, my career, social life, family life, and therefore every other aspect of my life, will be negatively affected. Speaking only for myself, I cannot say that I value not stinking and not becoming ill differently. I'm guessing that we are on the same page.

So here's the question: Why is one so easily addressed and the other has the power to make us completely miserable?

To be honest, I can only speculate. Maybe it's because grooming is conditioned in us from a very early age. If we were never taught personal hygiene, for example, maybe teeth-brushing would be as much of a chore as packing a lunch to avoid eating fast food. Maybe we would spend more time in front of a computer instead of bathing, just as so many people spend time on social media instead of exercising. If you were taught as a child that exercise was a nonnegotiable part of your weekly routine, maybe you would feel sort of gross and incomplete if you skipped it, like the way you probably feel if you forget to brush your teeth.

It is also very likely that instant gratification comes into play. When you take a shower and brush your teeth, you have an immediate sense of accomplishment: You are clean. When you begin eating and exercising properly, it will take a few days, at the very least, to see any changes, and most people will not notice any tangible changes in the first week, some not even in the first two weeks. Most of us are not very good at taking the long view, delayed gratification.

In my opinion, our everyday maintenance is easy while healthy changes are hard because the former is methodical and the latter is emotional. You have never tried to take a shower and failed. The information most widely available regarding teeth-brushing is not dead wrong. And nobody ever looked in the mirror with tear-filled eyes because she was too dirty and didn't know how to get clean. Frustration, anger, sadness, self-loathing— your morning routine does not inspire these thoughts to arise in you.

The trick is to try to remove your emotions from the situation so you can get down to business and reach your goals, but this can be easier said than done when you are haunted by the ever-present notion that you might fail. Trust me, if you thought you faced a high probability of failure as you attempted to groom yourself, you would be quite emotional about it. You must reassess your reasons for believing that failure looms ominously in the shadows.

There are only two reasons that people fail: lack of good information and lack of motivation. You are holding the necessary information in your hand right now, so all you have to do is elevate your motivation to get healthy and fit to the same level as your motivation to avoid having wavy cartoon stink lines above your head in all your photos. At this juncture, using your imaginary balance scale to weigh almost anything against personal hygiene and grooming is pointless. Personal hygiene and grooming will win every fight in which survival is not an immediate concern (unless you are camping, where all bets are off).

I understand that getting fit and healthy will add a few new "chores" to your schedule, but this will not be an issue when you are as motivated to get them done as you are to get your current daily chores done. Let me give you an example. Let's say you somehow offended a Zulu witch doctor, and he cast a spell on you that made you stink horribly unless you showered twice a day, once in the morning and once in the evening. What would you do? Well, you might not be ecstatic about it, but you would shower twice a day because stinking horribly is much worse. Simply put, you would weigh the options, consciously or not, and go with the option that most motivated you.

I am sure you can see where I am going with this. If you are serious about getting healthy and fit, eating and exercising properly *must* be added to the list of things you do without batting an eye. When it is simply part of your everyday life, Paleo will no longer be something you are "trying" any more than brushing your teeth would be described as a hobby you were trying.

I can't provide you with the motivation you will need. Nobody can. But hopefully you are starting to realize that there are no mysteries. You have been given all the information you need; your own desires will call the shots. If you don't reach your goals, it means that you clearly value the perceived benefits of your current lifestyle more than you value the potential benefits you would gain by changing. Where you place your values is entirely up to you, but there is no room for argument in that last sentence. From here forth there are no valid excuses. Your convictions are laid bare.

# High Stakes Done Right

Let's be realistic for a moment: You may never be able to give up on your aesthetic goals entirely, and that is perfectly fine. As long as you understand that you must get there by pursuing better health, you have my support. Change goals like "I want a smaller butt" to something like "I want to feel like a million bucks, even if it means a lot of hard work." That's all I am asking.

As we have already discussed multiple times, the reason your goals may remain elusive is that other things in your life are taking precedence over your desire to get healthy and fit, and this is probably even more true when immediate gratification is added as a factor in your decision-making. You might say to yourself, "I will just eat fast food this one time and then I will go right back to Paleo. It will only set me back a day." The problem is that you have set the stakes too low—there are no perceived consequences for getting off-track.

To see high stakes in action, we need only find someone with a deadline who is seriously desperate. Weddings and class reunions often provide the necessary stimulus. With a deadline and a perceived panel of judges, like wedding guests and former classmates, I have seen people go to lengths that even they had to think were insane. Caloric restriction on a massive scale, daily cardio/cortisol festivals, and strange supplements and shake concoctions are all the norm. And of course we can't leave out the holy grail of desperation, the cleanse, which is usually just starvation with a grander name. I have never known anyone to lose weight for a specific occasion and then keep the weight off. Again, I said "weight," not "fat," because none of those weight-loss tricks that seem so logical when you are desperate ever make you healthier. Remember, if a loss of mass does not make you healthier, it is not sustainable.

Isn't it funny how we can turn into complete lunatics when we feel like we will be on display? The intensity of motivation these events can conjure in us is astounding. If only that motivation were not misguided. What if you had all the right guidance *and* unwavering determination?

I would like to set a challenge before you, should you be so bold as to accept it. Here are the rules:

1. Choose at least five people to hold you accountable and ask them if they will be your panel of judges. A minimum of two of those people must not be related to you. You must choose at least five because we

all know two or three people who would never judge us harshly. If you have a mother who would tell you that you are beautiful after losing a heavyweight-boxing match, leave her out of this. This challenge will work best if you choose people you really like and respect and would also not want to let down. Ask everyone to help you reach your goals by not cutting you any slack.

2. Send everyone on your list "before Paleo" photographs, front and side angles, of you wearing nothing more than shorts and a tank top. Do not include your weight or any measurements.

3. Three months later, send them two more photographs, front and side angles, in the same clothes and with the same lighting.

4. After three more months (six months from your start date), send them two more photographs, front and side angles, in the same clothes (unless it would require duct tape to keep them on at this point) and with the same lighting. Ask for honest feedback comparing your three-month photographs with your six-month photographs.

5. After another three months (nine months from your start date), send them two more photographs, front and side angles, in the same clothes and with the same lighting. Ask for honest feedback comparing your three-, six-, and nine-month photographs.

6. Repeat this process again three months later (one year from your start date).

I know what you're thinking. After all my talk about not setting aesthetic goals, why am I throwing a purely aesthetic challenge at you? Because you cannot succeed at this challenge using tricks and gimmicks. Tricks and gimmicks do not produce results that will hold up to scrutiny for a whole year. You may be able to starve yourself thinner for the three-month photos, but you will not be able to continue to starve yourself for six, nine, and twelve months. Proper Paleo nutrition and exercise, on the other hand, will continue to produce improvements in most people for the entire twelve months. If you do not have far to go, you may reach your goals before the year is up, but then maintenance will be a cinch.

I will admit that I am being a little sneaky here. In reality, your only option is to set goals related to actually improving your health and fitness. Setting goals based only on trying to look good in your photos will probably mean failure. Sustainable improvements are all that matter in a situation like this, and only healthy improvements are sustainable. Since healthy methods will be essential, I am banking on your learning to love yourself along the way. It will be difficult to return to your old perspective after working so hard, and for so long, at treating your body the way it deserves to be treated.

I am not delusional. I know what I am suggesting is scary as hell! But if you dare to accept my challenge, pick worthy people to be your judges, and then follow through, you will succeed. If success has escaped you in the past, it very well might be because the consequences of failure did not terrify you. Making the consequences scary will keep you motivated, and the extended length of the challenge will force you to stay on the Paleo path to better health. A challenge like this is not the only route to success, but it is a great way to ask yourself, "How bad do I want this?"

## Bonus Points for the Very Brave

If you have the guts and want to change your body in a huge way while simultaneously motivating a lot of people, post your photos on Facebook for the whole world to see. When your results are on display, there is a good chance that some of your friends and family will also be inspired to change. You just might be a hero!

# CHAPTER 14
## game day jitters

## What's the Holdup?

If you're on the fence, you are not alone. Many people get stuck before starting. There may be other reasons for indecisiveness about Paleo, but the ones I'm going to mention are quite common and worthy of discussion. If you are overwhelmed by all the changes before you, flip back to the Slow Start section on page 161 and review your options. Otherwise, read on and allow me to challenge you to come down off that fence.

## Losing Streaks

You may have failed to reach the same health and fitness goal many times in the past. Or you may have lost and regained the same ten or twenty pounds multiple times. Either way, your fear of another failure may be keeping you from starting. If this is you, I have some advice for you from an unlikely source.

Tommy Angelo, author of *Elements of Poker*, has this to say about streaks:

*All of my good streaks and all of my bad streaks of every length and depth have had one thing in common. They did not exist in your mind. They only existed in my mind. And this is true for everyone's winning and losing streaks. None of them actually exist. They are all mental fabrications, like past and future. Everything that ever happens happens in the present tense. But how can you have a "streak" in the present tense? You can't. And therefore, if you are in the present tense, which, in fact, at this time, you are, then at this moment there is no streak in your life. There is no inherent existence to streaks. The streak is there when you think about it, and when you stop thinking about it, it goes away. It blossoms and withers, all in your mind. And when your mind invents a streak, you believe it exists, because you believe what your mind tells you. But the truth is there is only the hand you are playing.*

I really love Angelo's wisdom here. He may have been writing for poker players, but his wisdom applies perfectly to the limits some of us place on ourselves when it comes to our health and fitness goals. Your past efforts have no bearing on the present moment. You had bad information and things didn't work out. Forget about it. You have good information now. The cards have been shuffled and redealt. You've got a brand-new hand. Get in the game and play to win!

## Disbelief?

Maybe you just can't quite get your head around the fact that most of what you have been taught is complete bunk. To you, my friend, I issue my favorite challenge. Do you think that anything I am suggesting would kill you in a month? If not, then eat strict Paleo for at least three weeks. If you see no benefit to the way you look, feel, or perform, put a brick through my window and tell everyone on Facebook that I am a scam artist. Also, be sure to come to one of my seminars and heckle me.

I would certainly not say that if I had not seen the results with my own eyes, time and time again. While other diets ask you to dupe your body into the illusion of health, Paleo actually delivers health, and it usually begins working its magic right away. I am not claiming that Paleo will give you the results you want immediately, but you will see enough improvements in your health and vitality within three weeks to know that you have finally found what you have been looking for.

Nothing is more frustrating for someone like me than the critic who has never tried Paleo. I am not interested in discussing anyone's theories about why Paleo would not work for them. You have to come at me with something more tangible than that. All I am asking is that you give it a shot. Even if your only motivation is to make me eat my words. Please, just give it a shot.

# *Analysis Paralysis*

Once in a while I meet someone who is a veritable expert on the subject of Paleo, but still has not personally adopted the lifestyle. These people are the extreme case and not too common, but I see lesser degrees of analysis paralysis on a regular basis. Analysis paralysis happens when absorbing more information takes precedence over actually applying the information for the purpose it was originally sought. I think it is a common pitfall with Paleo because Paleo is literally the antithesis of everything most of us have been taught. Once you start learning the truth, it almost feels as if you are surrounded by conspiracy.

As we know, "common knowledge" can be hard to un-brainwash out of yourself. You may find yourself reading Paleo books and blogs every spare moment, yet a little voice in some recess of your mind is still stammering, "But, but, but. ..."

Would you like to know what will quiet that little voice every time? Results. When you understand the basics, you are going to have to dive in. As exciting as the information can be, the rewards of the Paleo lifestyle are so much better.

I am not saying the information doesn't matter. If you are a geek like me, by all means, don't ever stop learning about this stuff. There will always be more to learn. If you keep at it, you will eventually have the knowledge to recognize bad science when you see it. You will understand enough about biochemistry and physiology to track down the answers you seek, even when nobody in the Paleo community has directly addressed that specific subject. You will never make silly mistakes again because your judgments will be spot-on. Nobody will be able to back you into a corner with uneducated drivel like, "Grains are good for you and everyone knows it!" And you will probably look at your whole world through different eyes.

Yes, information is wonderful—just make sure you remember why you wanted it in the first place. As I said before, it is rare for anyone to become a Paleo expert without following through with action, but any time at all is too long to wait when you have absolutely nothing to lose except body fat, feeling bad, and an unhealthy relationship with a few bad foods.

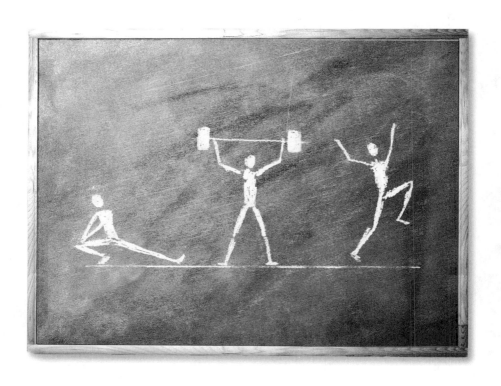

# MOVE

# CHAPTER 15
## *training to win*

### *Exercise: The Paleo Perspective*

We must move. All of us. The degree to which we move and the various ways in which we are capable of moving might be described as measures of our vitality, and vitality itself is a measure of how much we truly live, as opposed to merely exist. These truths have held true throughout humanity's time on earth, but we have lost sight of them.

To review, roughly 10,000 years ago, only a blip on our timeline, we wrested control from nature and began to grow our own food. Agriculture led to the world we live in today, with food always at our fingertips. In fact, it is so accessible that we barely have to interrupt our constant sitting position before we return to sit *and* eat. Unfortunately, this convenience is not part of the natural plan. For the majority of the 2.6 million years we spent becoming the creatures we are today, finding something to eat required movement. Sometimes a lot of movement. Thus, our bodies expect us to move. Yet we sit.

### *Diet <u>and</u> Exercise*

Some might disagree, but I refuse to consider the Paleo ideals without including exercise. If you want to achieve peak health, and you do if I have done my job well, exercise is a nonnegotiable part of the deal you will need to make with your body. Since you purchased this book and made it this far without tossing it into the fire, I will assume that you are on board with the idea that nutrition is important to your goals. Now you need to come to the same realization about exercising properly. Diet alone cannot deliver what you seek unless you set the bar much lower than I hope you will. As usual, I will not tell you what you should value, but I don't want you to misunderstand the implications that a sedentary life will have on your health and longevity. If you intend to follow the nutrition advice in this book, please remember that all of the people you will meet on these pages arrived at their successes through diet *and* exercise. This is not one of those commercials for a weight-loss pill that mentions exercise in the fine print at the bottom of your screen.

It is a sad truth that there are nutritionists in this world who do not understand exercise and trainers who do not understand nutrition. The simple fact that these subjects are separate at the academic level is a clear indication that the "experts" have long forgotten that the two are inextricably bound. While it is true that nutrition *or* exercise will usually bring about beneficial change for almost anyone the medical community would classify as "normal," to assert that either one alone can deliver peak health is fraudulent.

If you follow my logic and believe me when I tell you that exercise is essential to becoming as healthy as you can, then it is only a small step to believing that exercise makes all goals more attainable. Remember, regardless of your goal, success is sustainable only if your health is improved along the way. It may not feel like it at this exact moment, but your body wants you to exercise. Neglect to give it what it wants and it will do its best to adapt to the slower, squishier version of you that you are apparently intent on becoming. Just to make sure we are clear, I will state this fact as plainly as possible:

*If you want to be truly healthy, exercise is absolutely mandatory.*

If you have never exercised, you have some learning to do. If you have always exercised, there is a good chance that you have some unlearning to do. Either way, you can handle it, and the results are every bit as rewarding as getting your diet right. When you have a fit, capable body, not only will you feel amazing, but you will also have earned one more reason to stay on track. Physical accomplishments are hard earned. When you are proud of your strength and abilities, you will not want to let them be eroded by petty temptations. Junk food will never compare to the envy your friends will have as you coast through life's physical challenges without breaking a sweat.

Mainstream exercise advice is nearly as useless as mainstream nutrition advice, so some of what I am about to tell you might seem crazy. If you find yourself completely flabbergasted when you finish this section, I ask only that you humor me by taking the time to do it my way. Nothing I am going to share with you is untried or untested. Just give these methods an honest shot and see how you feel. What have you got to lose?

# Meander, Mosey, Stroll, and Saunter!

There are a few modalities of exercise that are indispensable. They are often overlooked, avoided, or underrated. One is walking. The first thing all beginning exercisers should do is increase the total amount of walking and low-intensity movement they do every day. This is especially true if you are a typical citizen of the Western world and the majority of your movement is to migrate yourself to another place to sit. I am not talking about strenuous exercise that leaves you tired and out of breath: I am referring to the type of physical activity that would have been your day to day routine if you sustained yourself by hunting and gathering.

If I show virtually anyone a picture of a lean, well-muscled hunter-gatherer and ask why that physique is the norm for people who live that way, I am invariably told that life is really hard for them and constant strenuous exercise keeps the fat off. This hypothesis is understandable considering the fact that so many of us have been sold on the notion that total hours spent exercising translates directly into total calories "burned," which translates into total fat loss. By that logic, more exercise is always better, so hunter-gatherers must live a very physically demanding life for obesity to be so rare among them. In reality, many anthropologists tell us that typical hunter-gatherers "work" an average of fifteen to twenty hours a week, with "work" consisting of a lot of walking.

According to anthropologist Frank Marlowe, who studied the Hadza people, modern-day hunter-gatherers in Tanzania, the women walk an average of just under three and a half miles per foray and men an average of just over five miles per day in their quest for food. Then there is the time spent performing other tasks, like gathering firewood and water. Therefore, even though they do not spend as many hours working as we do, they spend a lot more time engaged in low-intensity physical activity than most of us.

I am not suggesting that we all quit our jobs and head into the woods to scare up food every morning, but we cannot use our bodies in a manner so diametrically opposed to the way nature intended us to use them and expect to suffer no consequences. If a lot of low-intensity movement was required for survival for a couple of million years, our bodies became adapted to that movement. The negative impact of our huge reduction in low-intensity movement is not powerful enough to, say, render us infertile or kill us before we can reproduce; we are simply getting sick and dying before we should. No, I am not implying that walking is the cure for Western diseases or that not walking is the cause of all that ails us, but it is certainly another example of how ill-adapted our bodies are to the modern world we live in.

Maybe you already have a job that allows you to move around all day. If so, good for you. If not, get moving as often as you can each day. On the days when you can make the time, get out there and walk for half an hour or more. On busy days, one brisk ten-minute walk is a far cry better than nothing, and two or three such walks whenever you can fit them in would be fantastic. Walking is perhaps the one activity about which you can say that more is always better: some walking is better than none, and you really can't walk too much unless it causes you to miss a lot of meals or PTA meetings. There is also no need to huff and puff. If you can't hold a conversation while you walk, you are pushing yourself too hard. I'm not going to tell you exactly how much you should walk each week: Just walk whenever you can, understanding that that means *when you have time*, not *when you feel like it*.

This is also perhaps the only activity for which tricks and gimmicks really work: Parking farther away from the store is a great way to put in some extra pedi-miles; taking the stairs instead of the elevator is another great way to squeeze a little extra exercise into your day. If the weather where you live does not always cooperate, it's fine to jump on the treadmill. In fact, you can do almost anything that would be classified as "cardio," as long as it is done at approximately the same effort as walking. Faster is not better! (More on that in a moment.)

Once you are healthy and fit, walking will not feel like work, which is probably why it is ignored by so many people, including trainers, as a viable and necessary means of exercise. I really don't care how it's labeled as long as it gets done. If you are an athlete in impeccable physical condition, you should still find time to walk. If holding this book is the maximum amount of exercise you have done in years, walking is a great place to begin moving again. Make the time to get up and walk as if your life depends on it—because it just might.

# Pick Some Stuff Up!

Along with walking, resistance training—a.k.a. lifting weights—is right up there at the top of the list of indispensable modalities of exercise that everyone should be doing regardless of his goal. If you want to gain muscle, you should be lifting weights and walking. If you want to lose fat, you should be lifting weights and walking. If you want to get really healthy, you should be lifting weights and walking. If you want to live a long time, you should be lifting weights and walking. Do you see a pattern here?

I may have had you hook, line, and sinker when I told you to walk, but you might be squirming in your seat now that I mentioned weightlifting. I'm sorry to sound sexist, but it has been my experience that more women will balk at this advice than men. This is unfortunate because women are usually more passionate about changing the appearance of their bodies than men, and nothing returns better results in less time than lifting weights. Women, we will address your concerns shortly. Men, you may be just as guilty of avoiding resistance training, but for different reasons than women, which we will also cover soon. Let me go over the basic concepts first, and then we can talk about how to get everybody lifting.

There are many reasons that you should want to be strong and well muscled. (We can say "toned" if "well muscled" sounds too scary.) To name a few big ones, total muscle mass and base strength have been positively correlated to longevity over the last few decades; muscles increase metabolism, which makes it far easier to get and stay lean; and strength and power are the big drivers behind your capacity to work and play. Basically, if you want to live a long time in a body that looks and feels great, lifting weights will be a big part of how you get there. Does this advice sound like the opposite of everything you have always believed? Then it fits right in with the rest of my advice. Don't stop trusting me now! Every single person I train spends more of his or her time resistance training with me than anything else I ever have him or her do. This is true for men and women, from teenagers to seniors. Lifting is where it happens, whatever *it* may be.

Free weights are the way to go. Machines, while easy to use, are not a good replacement for barbells and dumbbells because they tend to work within very specific ranges of motion that eliminate the need for stabilization. So your prime mover muscles get strong but not your stabilizing muscles, which keep you from hurting yourself when you lift objects in your real life outside the gym. Even if your goals are purely aesthetic, and I hope they are not, you are selling yourself short if your training does not make your real-life physical activities easier. Free weights may require a better understanding of proper form and technique, but they also breed functional strength.

OK, here's the tricky part. This may not be what you want to hear, but the big compound (multi-joint) exercises—like the squat, dead lift, shoulder press, and bench press—are the most important of all the lifts. They train the body through natural movement patterns that we have all been do-ing for all of our lives. "What?" you may say. "I have never done a single dead lift!" Actually, you technically perform a dead lift every time you pick something up off the ground, but you probably do it with bad form, re-cruiting muscles in the wrong order and compromising your joints. The same can be said for squatting. Many doctors advise their patients never to squat to a full depth, in which the thigh is below parallel to the floor. Those doctors should have long ago starved to death in their bathrooms because a full squat is required for most of us to get off the toilet. Pushing objects requires the movement patterns used in the bench press, and lifting anything overhead, even a light bulb, requires a shoulder press. I am not saying you need to aim for the world record in these exercises, but if you must do them in real life, learning to do them correctly, safely, and with ease simply makes good sense.

Pull-ups and chin-ups deserve their own mention. They are not techni-cally *weightlifting* exercises, but they are very powerful resistance-training exercises that definitely translate well into real life. Pull-ups (palms facing away from you) and chin-ups (palms facing toward you) simulate how the upper body works when you climb, and maintaining your ability to climb might save your life someday. If you are like most beginners, pull-ups and chin-ups can seem impossible and, therefore, not worth further consider-ation. Don't worry—there is hope. Many gyms have weight-assisted pull-up machines that allow you to subtract a portion of your body weight from the total weight you need to pull with your arms. In my gym, we use resistance bands, like giant rubber bands, tied to our pull-up bars so clients can place a foot in the loop and use the elasticity of the band to help them complete pull-ups and chin-ups. Using these aids, virtually everyone can do a chin-up eventually, and a pull-up soon follows. As I write this, two women in my gym, Deb and Debbie (featured in the Never Too Old section, page 231), who are over fifty can do strict pull-ups, and neither ever did a single pull-up when she was under fifty. If you think they walked into my gym with the faintest inkling of ever doing a pull-up, you are sorely mistaken.

Up until now I have tried my hardest to make every step of your journey as easy as possible. I have given you options wherever I could that would allow you to take baby steps if that is what you need to get started. Unfortunately, I can't make this part much easier for you. You can start with body-weight exercises, but eventually you will have to lift weights three or four times a week in an organized manner, and that means you are going to need some education. I would love to be the coach who shows you the ropes, but proper lifting technique for beginners is way beyond the scope of this book. If you come to Everyday Paleo Lifestyle and Fitness (www.eplifefit.com), we will be happy to teach you proper form in intimate detail through demonstration videos and your own video submissions for critique. I know that sounds like a shameless plug, but I don't have a precise method for helping you find a good trainer, although I will do my best before we are done.

You don't have to make a lifetime commitment to personal training, and there is no need to spend thousands of dollars. You simply need an expert to teach you the basics so you can continue on your own. If you continue by yourself, I recommend that you check back in with us or your trainer once in a while to make sure you are still on track, but paying for a personal trainer doesn't have to be a regular expense. As with walking, you are going to have to take some initiative here. Get out there and learn to lift. I am asking you to trust me again. You will experience rewards beyond measure when you take my advice and get strong.

## Strength and Muscle Mass

It is probably safe to say that you have at least heard of bodybuilding. It is the type of competition (sport?) that Arnold Schwarzenegger made famous in which the goal is to achieve maximum muscle mass coupled with the best possible symmetry. The top bodybuilders in the world accumulate unbelievable amounts of muscle mass. If you have never seen a professional bodybuilder up close, they are quite impressive.

There is also a good chance that you have heard of powerlifting. Strength is the goal for powerlifters. Their competitions are won by the men and women in each weight class who lift the most weight in the back squat, dead lift, and/or bench press. These athletes are a true testament to what the human body can do with the right training and unwavering dedication.

Why are we talking about bodybuilding and powerlifting? Because it is important to note that these two types of competitions are not won by the same competitors. The top bodybuilders in the world are not the top power-lifters, and vice versa. In other words, the guys packing the most muscle are not the strongest men in the world, and the strongest men in the world are not packing the most muscle. If this all seems logical to you, then it should seem *illogical* to assume that muscle mass directly equals strength.

Many people assume that training with weights always means making muscles as big *and* strong as possible. If this were true, the winner of the world series of bodybuilding, the Mr. Olympia contest, would also hold all the powerlifting world records. To my knowledge, this has never happened, and it certainly has never happened in my lifetime. The training methods used by bodybuilders to build outrageous amounts of muscle are very different than the methods powerlifters use to develop muscles that are strong enough to lift outrageous amounts of weight. Typically, body-builders do three to five sets of eight to twelve repetitions of multiple exercises per muscle group, usually employing movements that isolate individual muscles in every workout. I'm sure there are plenty of bodybuilders who have other training strategies, but these parameters are the widely agreed upon basics of hypertrophy training, or training to increase muscle mass. Powerlifters, on the other hand, tend to perform lots of sets of very few, very heavy reps, with one to five reps being fairly standard. Training techniques do vary from athlete to athlete and workout to workout, but these are the general rules of thumb.

I realize that you probably are not setting your sights on the bodybuild-ing or powerlifting stages, but the take-home message for you is that your goal will determine how you train, and you do have a choice. If you want to get as big as you can, you will train to facilitate that goal. If you want your strength to be the stuff of legend, you will use the tried-and-true methods of those who have gone before you. Therefore, when I recommend that everyone get strong, relative to "normal," I am not at all insinuating that you should also want to be a behemoth. Strength and muscle mass are correlated, but they are not the same thing. *Capisce?*

# CHAPTER 16

## nobody is exempt from training

### Women and Muscle

Ladies, it's time to break your fear of weights. Almost every female member of my gym began her relationship with us by expressing her fear of amassing big muscles and looking like a man. I usually respond by saying that roughly 70 percent of our women dead lift 200 pounds or more, regardless of age. Then we walk out onto the workout floor, and I watch her looking around trying to find all the enormous he-women I just mentioned. She never finds any because we have never created any enormous he-women, despite the fact that we use a biased-protocol training method that is designed to increase maximum strength.

Take a look at this female bodybuilder.

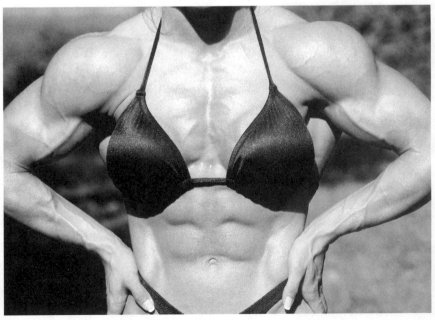

*Female Bodybuilder,* © *Hisham Ibrahim-Corbis*

Make no mistake: I am absolutely not passing judgment on anyone who actually wants to look like this. In fact, I have nothing but respect for the amount of work this woman put into her sport. But this required an unbelievable level of dedication to her very specific goal. To assume that your body might see even a fraction of these results by accident is insulting to female bodybuilders. This woman used training methods designed specifically for maximum muscle mass gain, tweaked every minute detail of her diet to help grow more muscle, and probably ate more food per meal than you eat all day. Do you intend to do *all* of those things? No? Then you can't look like her and worrying about it might be preventing you from being all that you can be.

In my experience, the women who can lift the heaviest weight and have the best overall physical capacity are also the women whose bodies elicit envy in everyone else. I think that most women who are new to fitness would assume that you can either be strong or you can be cute. I think most men would disagree—at least the men with any fitness experience.

Katie has been a client of mine for just over four and a half years, and she is pure awesome. On her first day of training she was a size 12 at 5 foot 2 inches. She is a mom with two young children, was eating the Standard American Diet, could barely do a sit-up, and was not happy with her body. This is what she looked like:

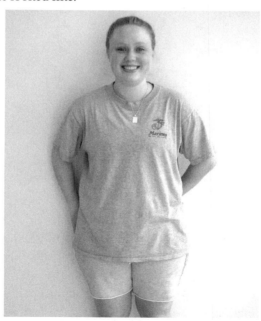

*Katie on her first day at my gym*

After deciding that she was fed up with her body, she got down to business with her training and nutrition and here are a few of her current stats:

Dead Lift: 260 lbs.
Back Squat: 200 lbs.
Shoulder Press: 85 lbs.
Bench Press: 105 lbs.

The average woman on the street is not likely to see numbers like these and think, "Wow, how very cute and ladylike." Aspirations of huge barbell lifts are not commonly associated with feminine behavior. But maybe they should be. You be the judge. Here is Katie at a size 4:

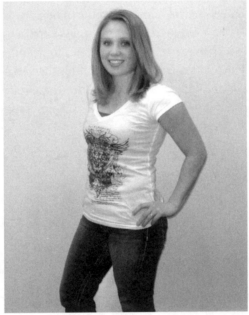

*Katie after some serious weight lifting*

The body you are looking at is the body that set all those personal records. As Katie got stronger, Katie got smaller. Her results are typical of all of my heaviest lifting women. Granted, they are not being trained exclusively for strength, and that is not what I'm recommending, but they are absolutely trained with strength and power as a top priority. In fact, when the newbies ask for advice from the top women, they are often told to get into lifting and get strong. I have no doubt that Katie would advise the same.

If I have not yet sold you on lifting weights, I have one more card to play. Other than the fact that weight training is key if you want to fast-track your goals, there is one more reason that all women could benefit from lifting. Bone density and osteoporosis. The only advice most women have been given to address this issue is to supplement with more calcium. The use of supplements always needs to be scrutinized. While some supplements are definitely beneficial, a great many that have claimed to be an antidote for the terrible way we treat our bodies have resulted in more problems. Calcium is no exception. While many studies have shown that calcium supplementation provides a bit of protection against bone loss, it has also been implicated in an increased risk of heart attack. A 2011 study titled "Calcium Supplements with or without Vitamin D and Cardiovascular Events: Reanalysis of the Women's Health Initiative Limited Success Dataset and Meta-analysis" had this to say in its conclusion:

> *Calcium supplements with or without vitamin D modestly increase the risk of cardiovascular events, especially myocardial infarction. ... A reassessment of the role of calcium supplements in osteoporosis management is warranted.*

I am only speculating here, but I think calcium supplements are going out of style. So, if calcium supplementation is beginning to get a bad rap, where do we go from there? We lift heavy things! In the Italian study "Effects of High-Intensity Resistance Exercise on Bone Mineral Density and Muscle Strength of 40- to 50-Year-Old Women," researchers concluded:

*These results suggest that even a short-term weight training program can either maintain or improve the BMD* (bone mineral density) *of the femoral neck and lumbar vertebrae in premenopausal women.*

One more and we can move on. For those of you who may be trying to ignore the word "heavy" every time I mention it, check out what the researcher had to say in the abstract of this study of postmenopausal women, the group with the highest risk of bone-mineral loss, titled "Exercise Effects on Bone Mass in Postmenopausal Women Are Site Specific and Load Dependent:

*Postmenopausal bone mass can be significantly increased by a strength regimen that uses high-load low repetitions but not by an endurance regimen that uses low-load high repetitions. We conclude that the peak load is more important than the number of loading cycles in increasing bone mass in early postmenopausal women.*

Translation: Five-pound dumbbells and a lot of repetitions will not solve the problem. You need to lift big, at least relative to your total strength.

Allow me one more attempt to appeal to you logically by asking a simple question: Have you ever met a woman who worked out with weights and got too muscular by accident? I am not asking about what you may have seen on TV, in movies, or any other media. I am asking if you know of a woman who built her muscles to an unfeminine level accidentally, without a ton of effort specifically aimed at maximum possible muscle mass. If your answer is no, and I'm sure it is, harboring a fear of getting too big has just stopped making sense. You have nothing to base this fear on because you have never seen it happen, not even once.

Please tell me that I have earned enough of your trust for you to at least try lifting weights for a couple of months. Find someone to show you how to move properly and stay safe, and then give it a go. I have introduced many women to weight training and have never heard a single regret. Try it. You'll see.

## The Quest to Build Giant Women

In an attempt to finally put down the fear many women have of getting too muscular and masculine, I asked for the help of a couple of clients who trust me. My idea was to spend three months training these women for maximum hypertrophy (muscle growth) and record their progress with photos. I presented my idea to Angela, whose story you read earlier, and Jen, who had already accomplished many of her physical-capacity goals in my gym. Both women agreed to participate and we got to work.

I wrote programs specifically designed to turn them into giant, muscle-bound Vikings. Their diets were tweaked to remove any shred of fat loss protocol, which included increasing their calories and starchy vegetable and fruit consumption. We also removed all huffing and puffing from their workouts, even in their warm-ups. In short, I threw everything I had at them, and they trained very much like professional female bodybuilders would in a mass gain phase, but without any performance-enhancing drugs.

This is what they looked like on day 1:

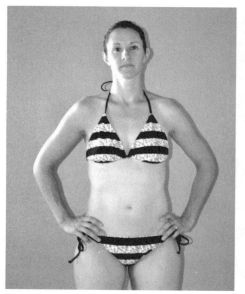

*Jen before picture*

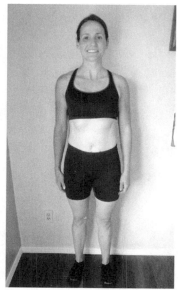

*Angela before picture*

And here they are at the end of the twelve-week experiment to get huge:

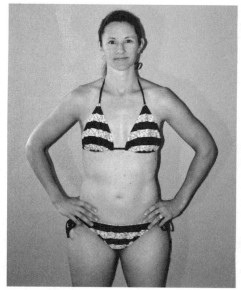

*Jen 12 week picture*

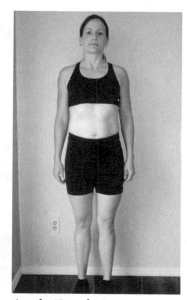

*Angela 12 week picture*

Just for fun, here they are in street clothes:

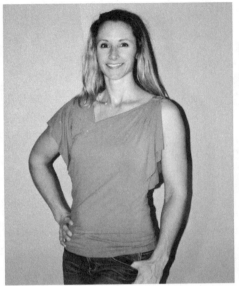

*Jen 12 week picture*                                  *Angela 12 week picture*

As you can plainly see, my experiment was a miserable failure. Neither woman was transformed into a silverback gorilla on steroids. In fact, by most standards, both women actually increased their attractiveness despite training in a fashion almost universally believed to make women less attractive.

I suppose it would've been possible for these ladies to have grown more muscle, maybe even manly muscles, if our experiment had been carried out over more time, but this is an irrelevant point. The common fear among women is that lifting weights will *accidentally* result in masculine muscles, and if three months of training specifically for muscle growth is not enough time to produce such results, it would appear that women cannot become victims of unwanted muscle mass because growing big muscles is a slow and deliberate process for women, if it happens at all. On the contrary, most women probably cannot grow masculine muscles, even if they really work at it, unless they have some chemical help.

All right, already, I'll put this subject to bed, but it should be quite obvious that I *really* want all the women reading this book to start training with free weights. If you give it a shot, I will consider it a personal victory, but it's not about me—it's about you! If our paths should ever cross, I would love hear all about your lifting exploits.

## *Men and Muscle*

Men, please forgive me for the brevity of this section compared with the effort I put into trying to convince the ladies to lift, but the idea of more muscles is a lot easier to sell to you. Most of us would like to be well defined and relatively lean. Since we come in different shapes and sizes, the end result of our efforts also comes in different shapes and sizes, and there are different paths to get there, depending on where we start. A complete lack of knowledge on this subject does not make you a girlie man, despite what Hanz and Franz told us on *Saturday Night Live*. There is no shame in a general disinterest in lifting weights up to this point. Just understand that you will need to get educated before you jump in. Don't let your pride get the better of you. It is much better to be seen working with a trainer than getting it wrong.

If you are naturally on the thin side, you probably don't have to worry too much about putting on fat, but building muscle is really tough. (For the ladies reading this section, stop telling these men that you envy them for being skinny! They don't want to be skinny, and it is tantamount to them telling you that you are fat.) If you are going to succeed in putting on some lean bulk, there are a couple of things you must wrap your head around.

First, you need to *eat*. If you are consuming fewer than 3,000 calories per day, you are not serious about gaining muscle; a minimum of 3,500 calories per day would be better. Pro bodybuilders put that to shame, and Olympic swimmer Michael Phelps says he eats 12,000 calories a day, but it would be really difficult to get there without eating a lot of garbage. Once you are consuming enough calories to fuel your mass-gain goal, just keep an eye on your results and tweak things as necessary. For example, if you start to put on more fat than you would like to see, try adjusting your carbs or condensing your eating window each day without reducing your calories. Just be sure to be patient and make one change at a time. Muscle mass is hard earned, and your progress will be slower than if your goal were fat loss.

Second, you need to lift heavy weights in lots of different ways and stop huffing and puffing in your workouts. If muscle mass is your primary goal, cardio is even more useless for you than it is for everyone else, but you also have no real need for high-intensity interval training (more on that coming up) or any other type of conditioning work. This is not to say that you can never do anything but lift weights, but a lot of training in various energy pathways will only negate some of the effort you are putting in by consuming all those calories. Your routine workouts should resemble bodybuilding workouts with some maximal-strength powerlifting thrown in. When the weights are lighter and the repetitions are in the mass-gain range of eight to twelve, keep your breaks short. On heavy days, rest as necessary between sets without letting yourself cool down.

If you are already a big guy, weight training will be a valuable tool to help you get healthy and lean, but you must remember that fat loss happens mostly at the table. Losing fat should be your first priority if you have a lot to lose. Building muscle may be easier for you than it is for your thinner counterparts, but massive muscles will not negate a lot of excess fat. Just imagine how wide your shoulders would have to be to give you a nice V shape if you have a big waist. Get your diet right, lift heavy, and count your lucky stars that there will be muscles under there when Paleo has worked its magic. Those of us who are hard gainers envy the ease with which you pack on muscle. You also have the advantage of being able to focus your training largely on your performance goals if you so desire. You can train for strength, muscle mass, or conditioning and general fitness, and whatever you choose, you will still lose fat if your diet is right.

No matter who you are or how you are built, don't forget that improved health is the first consideration for any goal. Eating junk to fuel your gains may actually help you get bigger, but at what cost? Weight-loss tricks and gimmicks may actually reduce the number on the scale, but is that number sustainable? As men, we endure fewer societal pressures regarding the way we look than women do, but we are no less guilty of doing the ridiculous to reach our goals.

## Lifting in the Gym

Now that you understand how important it is to lift weights, you will either need access to a gym or you will have to buy some equipment. In my opinion, joining a gym is better. The workout floor at your local gym will not be ten steps from your couch, as it would be if you set up a gym in your garage. Going to the gym will mean entering a facility specifically designed for working out, and the distractions will be far fewer than in your home with all its comfortable spots for being lazy. But you may decide the gym is too scary and never join. So let's think it through.

It is quite common for people to think they are not fit enough to go to the gym. The reasoning is that there are fit people there and not being fit might make a person stand out. This is kind of like saying, "I am way too sick to go to the doctor. I need to get over this virus before I go because there might be people there who aren't as sick as me." How do you improve your fitness? You work out. Where do you go to work out? The gym. So, what happens at gyms? People work out and improve their fitness. Therefore, we can assume that people who join gyms are looking for only two things: the acquisition of new fitness or the maintenance of fitness already acquired. Are you as fit as you would like to be? No? Then where should you go? That's correct, to the gym. If the gym is *the* place to go to get fit, fabricating an entry-level fitness standard in your mind is only self-defeating. You will only be preventing yourself from going somewhere that other people go to find exactly what you are looking for.

Those people at the gym whose judgment you may fear, the already fit people, are not better than you; they simply got there first—they have been working on their fitness for a while. They don't have superpowers and they are not from royal bloodlines with a distaste for commoners like you and me. They are just people working on their fitness. In fact, if you hang out at any gym long enough, you will get to know some of those people, and you will be glad to see them when you arrive for your workout.

There is one particular creature found on the weight floor of some gyms, and he can be a bit annoying if you acknowledge him. Commonly known as a "Bro," he is a very special kind of gym rat whose identity is attached to the number of hours he spends staring at his body in the mirror in front of the dumbbell racks. This ritual is often followed by plenty of time scanning the gym in the hope that other people are equally admiring his body. The Bro is easily ignored, and legend has it that he will eventually turn to dust and blow away if nobody looks at him. This is why Bros often travel in packs. Having other Bros around to admire each other's bodies helps reduce the risk of disintegration.

All joking aside, there is nobody in any gym anywhere who should ever be given the power to keep you from improving your health and fitness. The opinions of others will never amount to anything other than the value you assign to them, and your goals have far more inherent value, if only because they are *yours*. You do not want to lie on your deathbed with the knowledge that things could have been better if you had not spent so much time making assumptions about what total strangers might be thinking. Get in there and get to work, and to hell with your destructive inner voice.

# CHAPTER 17
# get fast and stay loose

## What Are You Running From?

When we watch young mammals at play, we tend to see behavior that mimics hunting, escaping, and mating rituals. Why? Because play is practice for real life. Our kids play instinctively. We don't need to teach our kids how to play. Taking them to a playground is enough—they are perfectly capable of figuring the rest out on their own. They wrestle, climb, jump, swing, sprint, roll, dodge, crawl, pick stuff up, throw stuff, and catch stuff. But when we open our front doors to let our kids go outside, do they ever take off on a three-mile run? No? Weird. They are not instinctively driven to run long distances because doing so will not make them better at hunting and gathering.

Cardio is a strange concept. Somehow it has become the gold standard for exercise, even though it doesn't seem to be working for anyone. Think about it. There are really only two types of bodies at marathons: the emaciated bodies of the hardcore runners and the still-squishy bodies of those who think running is a good way to lose fat. Neither of those body types is anyone's goal. The emaciated types are often fine with their bodies because they run for sport and being light can be an advantage, but they are not running for their health any more than football players play football for health. All the other runners have been led to believe that running is a good way to get healthy and fit, despite the fact that steady-state cardio offers no survival advantage in humans and is therefore not a form of movement to which we are adapted.

Sprinting makes perfect sense to our bodies. The ability to run very quickly over a short duration is the ability to escape predators and catch food. Hormones like adrenaline and cortisol help facilitate maximum-effort sprints when necessary. Unfortunately, our bodies do not expect us to run long distances for no reason, and the hormones that respond are the same whether we jog ten miles or sprint fifty yards. Basically, cardio produces the stress response that is the result of our bodies going, "Please let me escape this unbelievably persistent tiger!" This state of stress, marked by a cortisol spike, is not conducive to losing fat while maintaining muscle and staying healthy. The outcome is emaciated muscles and midsection fat that hangs on for dear life because your body does not want to let go of its emergency energy stores during this time of constant stress. If you run for sport, I have absolutely no qualms with you. You have other goals besides fat loss and peak health, and I get it. Nobody plays professional football to get really healthy and live a long time, either. Everyone else, you need to rethink all that cardio.

Whenever I meet a young man with a newfound interest in bodybuilding, he always has a hero or two from the monstrous competitors. He may never amass the amount of muscle his heroes have, but every step between here and there will mean more muscle. Running works the same way, but nobody takes this into consideration. The most elite distance runners have lost so much muscle mass that nobody would mistake them for healthy-looking individuals, and doing what they do is the best way to get what they have. I think too many people probably assume they can stop short of that extreme at a *weight* that is desirable. This is a clear indication of some of the problems we talked about in the first half of this book. Getting to a lighter weight at any cost does not improve attractiveness because it does not improve health.

If you have a lot of weight to lose, cardio can seem like the way to go because it does make people smaller, but you should be aiming for the body you truly want and not just a smaller version of the one you have. If you know someone who lost a lot of weight predominantly through lots of cardio, did he really end up with a good body? Probably not. Small and squishy might be better than big and squishy, but healthy and toned is comfortable in a bathing suit.

Enough logic. Let's talk science. The title of this study says it all: "Two Minutes of Sprint-Interval Exercise Elicits 24-Hour Oxygen Consumption Similar to That of 30 Minutes of Continuous Endurance Exercise." Oxygen consumption is where fat loss happens. This study compared the fat-loss benefits of two minutes of sprint intervals with thirty minutes of standard cardio and found them to be approximately equal. Consider this statement from the abstract:

*Despite large differences in exercise $VO_2$ (oxygen uptake at the muscles), the protracted effects of SIE (sprint interval exercise) result in a similar total*

*$VO_2$ over 24 hr vs. CEE (continuous endurance exercise), indicating that the significant body-fat losses observed previously with SIT are partially due to increases in metabolism postexercise.*

Translation: Two minutes of sprinting results in the same capacity for fat loss as thirty minutes of cardio when measured over a twenty-four-hour period, except without all the excess stress. Therefore, cardio for fat loss is nothing more than a huge time suck with side effects that are quite effective at negating the reasons anyone would do cardio in the first place.

OK, so sprinting is great, but what does it look like for the average, non-track star, person? It is really quite simple, because sprinting effort is subjective—it depends on your own fitness. In other words, I'm sure I will be sprinting when I'm eighty, but it will probably look a little different than it does now. No matter, 100 percent effort is all it takes, regardless of the outcome.

My favorite way to introduce beginners to sprint intervals is on a track. Start by warming up thoroughly with some walking and light jogging, maybe alternating between the two once around the track. Then find something to hold on to and swing one leg at a time, front to back, through a full range of motion to warm up your hamstrings and hips. You could also throw in some plyometric movements like jumping jacks or burpees. When you feel warmed up, especially your hamstrings and calves, you are ready to begin.

Simply walk briskly around the track and sprint one of the two straight sections each time you come to it. For example, you might start walking at one of the turns, continue through the back straight section and through the second turn, and then run as fast as you can through the front straight section back to the first turn, where you return to your brisk walk. Do this four times and you will have covered approximately one mile (on a standard 400 meter track), with four sprints mixed in and plenty of time to catch your breath in between. If you stick to a good pace on the walks, the whole workout will probably take you less than fifteen minutes. If you are not quite ready to sprint that far, just go as far as you can each time. It is also a good idea to complete your first sprint at a submaximal level, maybe 70 or 80 percent of all-out effort, just to make sure you get fully warmed up.

Of course, sprints can be done in less time by walking only until you catch your breath and then immediately sprinting again. They can also be done wherever you can find the space to do them. There is no need to ever go more than one mile in the entire workout, and you should incorporate sprints into your routine once or twice a week. Mark Sisson, author of *The Primal Blueprint*, likes to do his sprints on the beach. If you want a real challenge, do your sprints on stairs, and you will definitely remember the workout the next day. Rowing machines and exercise bikes are good options when getting outdoors isn't possible, but try to mix them up. Treadmills are not a good idea because they don't allow for maximum acceleration. Whatever you do, stop doing steady-state cardio for fat loss and start doing things that actually make you better at being a human.

## Cardiorespiratory Workouts Designed for Humans

There is another way, besides sprints, to train for improved conditioning and cardiorespiratory endurance. In high-intensity interval training (HIIT), intensity, defined by total effort, varies intermittently from very high to moderate or low. For fat loss and general health goals, HIIT can be a valuable tool to add to an exercise regimen in which lifting and walking are already firmly established. If you are not lifting and walking as you should be, get on them first.

Probably the most famous study on HIIT, conducted by researcher Izumi Tabata in 1996, is "Effects of Moderate-Intensity Endurance and High-Intensity Intermittent Training on Anaerobic Capacity and $VO_2$ Max." One group of subjects trained on exercise bikes at 70 percent of maximal oxygen uptake, a good midrange intensity for typical cardio, for sixty minutes a day, five days a week, for six weeks. A second group trained on exercise bikes using HIIT. Intervals consisted of twenty seconds at as much as 170 percent of $VO_2$ max (very high effort!), followed by ten seconds of rest, for a total of eight cycles. This means they were working very hard for twenty seconds, resting for 10 seconds, until they had completed the cycle eight times in four minutes. After both groups were tested, researchers reported the following:

*In conclusion, this study showed that moderate-intensity aerobic training that improves the maximal aerobic power does not change anaerobic capacity and that adequate high-intensity intermittent training may improve both anaerobic and aerobic energy supplying systems significantly, probably through imposing intensive stimuli on both systems.*

Translating from geek speak, this study showed that endurance training (standard cardio) improves only aerobic capacity, which is about endurance, while HIIT improves aerobic capacity *and* anaerobic capacity, which is how strength and muscle mass are improved. It's like killing two birds with one stone in far less time than it takes to plod down the road with that look of misery so common on the faces of runners.

HIIT is great, but I have a few words of warning for you. First and foremost, do not overdo it! I understand that working out in a fashion that smashes you and leaves you sucking wind on the floor can fill you with pride and a sense of accomplishment, but it can also lead you to believe that more is better. It's not. Twenty-minute HIIT workouts should be rare, unless the intensity is not actually high, and thirty-minute HIIT workouts are no longer HIIT workouts—they are just crazy. The result of overtraining with HIIT is adrenal fatigue, which will slam the brakes on you, forcing you to take a long enough vacation from the gym to undo a lot of hard-earned progress and leave you with a long road to recovery from fatigue. If you employ HIIT in your exercise routine, be responsible by keeping the intensity high and the duration short. Remember, Tabata's subjects did only four minutes of intervals. Period. Try his exact workout sometime (twenty seconds at max effort plus ten seconds of rest times eight), and then see if you think you need more. Prepare to be shocked.

I already alluded to the second thing you need to know about HIIT, but it bears repeating. HIIT should not replace lifting and walking (or low-intensity movement) as your primary methods of training. In my opinion, HIIT is excellent but supplemental. Everyone should incorporate some HIIT into his regular routine, but not at the expense of lifting weights or low-intensity movement. Athletes are sometimes the one exception to this rule, depending on the demands of their sport. Therefore, everyone with health and fat-loss goals, which are really the same thing, should be lifting and walking before implementing HIIT. The reason I am trying to drive this point home is that many people, when left to their own devices, will skip lifting and walking in favor of huffing and puffing because the concept of cardio for weight loss has been forced upon them for so long that they just can't free themselves of it. Remember, you do not want *weight loss*, and *fat loss* happens almost entirely at the kitchen table.

So get your lifting and low-intensity movement dialed in, and then throw in a short sprint session once a week. When you've got all that running smoothly, turn up the intensity with some responsible HIIT. You don't need to do more than a total of three sprint workouts and HIIT workouts combined.

# Get Mobile!

If strength and power translate to our ability to do work and move ourselves through life, mobility defines our capacity to move without injury and/or pain. For our purposes here, mobility encompasses flexibility and range of motion as well as muscle imbalances. Often neglected, especially by men, mobility is another aspect of fitness that is completely nonnegotiable and absolutely necessary for everyone. Once you have learned how to acquire and maintain proper mobility in all of your joints, you will fully understand that the overwhelming majority of exercise-related injuries are avoidable.

It would require another entire book to fully educate you on all the various mobility techniques, so I am just going to give you a few basic pointers. But I am also going to point you to physical therapist and mobility guru Kelly Starrett, whose Web site is Mobility WOD (Workout of the Day); www.mobilitywod.com. The site is one gigantic compilation of short videos focusing on mobility in more ways than most people will ever have the time to entirely absorb. If you have a problem related to mobility, he has addressed it from a few different angles already, and videos are continually being added to the mix. Starrett's other major contribution to proper movement is his excellent book, *Becoming a Supple Leopard*, in which he leaves us guessing at nothing. His knowledge on the subject of mobility is much greater than mine, so I will refer you to him for further details, but there are some things you need to know right now.

Our modern lives put most of us in unnatural positions, like sitting in chairs for hours each day. As hunter-gatherers we would have rarely found opportunities to sit in the position you just may be in right now—feet on the floor, back supported. Nature doesn't often provide structures that allow us to assume such a position. Sitting like this tends to encourage rounding in the lower back and tightness and weakness in the hips. When we ask our bodies to sit, sit, sit, and then expect them to do work, we are asking for trouble. Back, knee, and hip pain are so common that it may be easier to count the adults in the Western world who do not suffer from any of these complaints. The truth is that, unless there is an accident resulting in injury, or another external input like poor nutrition, improper movement is to blame for aches and pains related to joints. For example, tight hip flexors, from sitting too much, often contribute to a forward-tilting pelvis (anterior tilt), causing extension in the low spine, which usually results in lower back pain. Since very few of us have the power to drastically alter the way we spend our days, we must make a concerted effort to keep our bodies moving as they should if we want to live pain free. If you are young and don't have any aches and pains, you may be tempted to skip this section. Trust me, proper mobility now will keep you from ever joining the ranks of those who are reading this section hoping for some relief.

No matter how tight and inflexible you have become, if you have not weathered any major reconstructive surgeries, you should be able to entirely recover the excellent mobility you had as a small child. But make no mistake, this will require constant effort through short daily sessions of mobility work that, in reality, is not very difficult to fit into your day. The good news is that nothing I have talked about or will talk about in this book has the potential to yield faster progress than mobility. I have seen people resolve pain they have dealt with for decades with less than a week of proper mobility work.

One concept that cannot be overlooked is balanced mobility. In my gym, almost everyone comes to us with muscle imbalances in which a muscle or group of muscles on one side of the body is tighter than the same muscle(s) on the other side of the body. This is absolutely not something to shrug off and chalk up to your individual quirkiness. Imbalances like these can be equated to driving your car when it is out of alignment, only instead of your mechanic selling you new tires, your doctor will sell you painkillers. If you find an imbalance, you should not continue to stretch both sides as far as they each will go because you will only perpetuate the muscle imbalance. Instead, stretch your tight side first and then match its range of motion on your more flexible side. Using the hamstrings as an example, you might sit down on the floor with your tighter leg straight and lean your torso toward it while reaching for your foot. If you are able to reach only the middle of your shin, this is as far as you should stretch on your more flexible side, even if you can go much farther. Stretching both sides with equal tension will potentially lengthen both sides equally, preserving the imbalance. In other words, if you lengthen both sides by one inch, the difference between the two sides will still be the same—they will simply both be an inch longer. Fixing muscle imbalances should be your top priority, and they get fixed by making strength and range of motion symmetrical.

As long as you are aware of your imbalances, the best advice I can give you on stretching is *do it*. Do it after every workout and on every day you don't work out. The only time you should not stretch aggressively is just before you work out. Muscles should be warmed up and ready to go before exercise, but save the serious mobility work for afterward. The exception to this rule is in situations in which extreme tightness in a specific muscle group prevents proper range of motion in a given movement. If your hips are too tight to squat properly and trying to do so compromises your low-back position, stretching your hips before squatting may help keep your back safe. In that case, stretch as necessary. Otherwise, post-workout stretching is best.

If you take my word for it and put some honest effort into acquiring better mobility, you will see results quickly enough to keep you motivated to continue. Then, when you are truly mobile, you will feel as if you are rolling on greased bearings and you will never let that feeling go.

# CHAPTER 18

## play smart to win

### Take a Break!

Here's a fun piece of trivia for you: You do not gain physical capacity or grow muscles in the gym. The only thing that happens in the gym is the application of various stimuli that elicit adaptation during rest and recovery. In plain English, our work in the gym causes us to gain strength, muscle mass, and/or overall fitness *during recovery*. It is important to understand this fact because the belief that more training is better has slowed or halted the progress of multitudes of motivated people. A lack of adequate recovery time between workouts leads to overtraining, and when overtraining stops you from making gains, you might think you aren't working hard enough, and so you work out even harder or longer or more often. This can turn into a nasty downward spiral resulting in adrenal fatigue or injury, not to mention an inability to reach your goals. You don't want to end up saying, "I worked my butt off and it still didn't work!" The process is train, recover, repeat. You will spin your wheels if you are always training and never recovering.

You can and should walk and stretch every single day, but lifting weights, sprinting, and high-intensity interval training should be confined to no more than four days a week for most people with fat loss and health goals. Approximately 90 percent of the members of my gym work out three days a week and not one time have we encountered a situation in which adding more workout days was the missing piece of the puzzle preventing someone from reaching his health and fitness goals. This is very often a hard concept for new clients to understand. Many of them tell us that they want to sign up for an unlimited membership and come five or six days a week. When we tell them that they can't work out more than three days a week to start, they are always perplexed. Of course, we are proud of them for their drive, but it's our job to help them understand that adequate recovery time is the fast track to success. We explain that we can reevaluate in the near future and add more days if necessary, but it has never been necessary and nobody ever asks to add more days.

I prefer that my clients never train more than two days in a row. If both weekend days are convenient for workouts, so be it, but then both Monday and Tuesday would best be used as rest days. Occasional exceptions can be made immediately before extended absences from the gym. For example, if you are going on vacation for a week or two, working out three days in a row before you leave will probably not kill you.

One of the key aspects of rest and recovery is to listen to your body. Try not to let dates and times alone dictate your workout schedule in any week. If you are exhausted and sore, you need to take a rest day, even if you already took one. Don't go to the gym and push yourself through a workout just because it is Wednesday and you always work out on Wednesdays. Also, don't consider only exercise-related stress when deciding whether or not to work out. Stress from work and relationships can negatively affect rest and recovery, causing a greater need for more space between workouts. For example, if you can't sleep because you are too stressed out about a project at work, an extra day off from the gym might be necessary. Your body will try to tell you when it needs a little more recovery time. Listening to it does not make you weak or unmotivated. Just be honest with yourself about when and why you rest.

Taking an entire week off every six to eight weeks of training is a fantastic idea for everyone. Personally, it seems as if life handles this for me most of the time, but I am always aware of how long it has been since I had some extended downtime just in case a forced break doesn't present itself. The first time you take a whole week off you may feel a little anxious about it. That sinister little voice in your head will be yelling, "You're losing everything you worked for!" Tune it out, as usual. You may be a little out of practice in your first workout when you return to the gym, but within that week you will feel as if you are firing on all cylinders again.

Strive for balance between working hard and recovering well. The greatest progress happens when ample rest follows exercise performed with adaptation in mind, which brings me to my next point.

# Intensity

Intensity is a tricky subject and challenging to teach. Controlling workout intensity, turning it up very high for short durations and knowing how high to keep it through a workout, is a learned skill for most people. Few people can walk into a gym for the first time and push themselves to the edge of their physical capacity. Yet this skill is the one thing that will allow you to get the most out of every workout without spending your whole life in the gym. It is best learned by example, but since I can't join you for your next workout, I will try to convey the key factors involved so that you can begin to experiment on your own.

In resistance exercise, intensity is defined by the amount of effort you put into completing difficult reps. A set in which you barely complete the final repetition is more intense than a set in which you stop short of that rep. In sprints and high-intensity interval training, intensity is defined by your ability to push yourself to do more work in less time. This is where the mental game comes in, because you really need to ignore your head and listen to your body.

When training new clients in my gym, we are almost always able to encourage inexperienced people to complete more reps than they thought they could. Their minds are saying, "This is really heavy and I want to stop now," but their muscles still have some gas in them. When they do finally put the weight down, they usually say something about how hard the set was, but it's always obvious that they are impressed with themselves for getting through it. Those first few workouts are an eye-opening experience for beginners because they get to find out what they are truly capable of doing.

We don't torture people and we are not sadistic, although I have certainly been accused of such behavior. The reason for keeping intensity high in most workouts is to elicit the maximum adaptation response while controlling stress as much as possible. And of course we don't want to waste time by spinning our wheels in the gym. The gist is this: Get in there and work really hard over a short amount of time if you really want success, rather than lackadaisically going through the motions like you are being forced to do something you hate.

A stopwatch can be handy when trying to increase intensity in sprints and high-intensity interval training because you'll know what time you have to beat next time. Intensity can go through the roof when you are trying to squeeze the same amount of work into less time and set a new personal record. However, bad form in exchange for a faster time is not acceptable. Being safe always trumps bragging rights, and even if you don't get hurt in a specific sloppy workout, don't assume that you haven't done any damage. Regularly performing any movement with improper form will teach your body to assume that same bad form each time you do that movement. We refer to this as *grooving bad movement patterns,* and it should be avoided at all costs. Form first, then intensity. Period.

We never yell or scream at people in my gym—we just give direction—so you don't really need me beside you as long as you can imagine me standing there saying, "Don't quit yet. You can do one more." Just understand that when you ask, "Can I keep going?" you are asking your powerful muscles, not your lazy brain. It may take some practice, but increasing the intensity in your workouts will lead to the rewards of reaching your goals faster and spending less time in the gym.

## The Stuff You Hate

It should now be clear that a good fitness routine, regardless of your goal, will include low-intensity movement, resistance training with free weights, sprint intervals, and mobility work. If you already love all of those things, you are a rare breed. Most of us like one type of training, don't really mind one or two, and hate one or two with every fiber in our bodies. Unfortunately, there is no room for emotion when it comes to an optimal exercise program. While it is important to have fun, sometimes you have to do the stuff you hate.

Personally, I really enjoy lifting weights in the repetition ranges that build muscle mass (eight to twelve reps per set), and I enjoy walking and hiking. I don't like being out of breath, and I have never really enjoyed maximal-strength training. However, I understand that achieving and maintaining excellent health and fitness means that sometimes my workouts must leave me sucking wind and that my strength needs to be far above the average for Western males my age. Therefore, I do not have a love affair with sprints and very heavy lifting, but I do them because the alternative is normal and normal is a far cry from acceptable.

We only tend to truly hate the things we do not do well. This is good news, because if we force ourselves to do them anyway, we will improve. For example, while I may not love sprinting, I don't hate it. I have spent enough time sprinting to recognize the rewards it delivers, and it has become a worthwhile component in my fitness routine. If I hated sprinting, I would have to grit my teeth to get through every sprint workout, having only narrowly escaped all the distractions that were more seductive. If I didn't tough it out in the beginning, I would probably not be sprinting today, and my overall fitness and health would suffer.

The takeaway is that having the discipline to do things outside your comfort zone will eventually decrease their discomfort. And who knows? You might even like them one day. Doing your best to focus on your accomplishments or goals instead of on your distaste for the task at hand can be a huge help when you are getting started. If you have a strong desire to avoid lifting weights, keep a notebook and track the weights you are using so you can celebrate each time those weights increase in any exercise. If you hate sprinting, start timing your sprints so you can try to beat your best time in your next sprint workout. (Rowing machines are great for this because they track your time and meters travelled.) However you do it, just get through the stuff you hate enough times for your inner voice to finally shut up when it realizes you are not going to quit. I am not suggesting that you have to become a world-class athlete—only that you give your body what it wants so it will return the favor. The only other option is to wallow in your comfort zone, and that is likely to leave you with subpar results—and you deserve more. Much more.

## No Time to Exercise?

Just like the argument that Paleo food is too expensive, the excuse of no time for exercise is valid—for a few people. I'll admit that life can get really crazy sometimes, but you are actually too busy to exercise only if you would have to stop bathing in order to do so. If your cleanliness is not at risk, you probably just need to summon some motivation. This is where your personal desire to reach your goals will come into play.

Adequate exercise for improving health, losing fat, and gaining muscle takes only two hours a week, or four half-hour sessions, with some walking thrown into the mix. If you told me that you truly want to be healthy and fit but don't have two hours a week to spare, I would have to assume that you don't have a Facebook account, a favorite TV show, or any hobbies. If you have these things and aren't willing to give them up in order to reach your goals, that's fine, but please understand that you have weighed these other activities against your fitness goals and have found your fitness goals wanting. You have to know where you stand, so be honest with yourself.

# Getting Back In the Game

Somewhere, at some time, you are going to experience some downtime. You are going to get sick, or go on vacation, or become temporarily overwhelmed with other demands in your life, and you will not be able to work out for a while. Trust me, it will happen, and it's fine. The only question that needs answering is, *What will you do when the downtime is over?*

I have seen a great many people become completely derailed by the psychological repercussions from downtime. They fear that their time off has robbed them of all their gains, and the thought of returning to their workouts is just too scary. Many of these people walk away from all their hard work, never to return. They look back with regret, not because they quit, but because they believe they would have been fine if only their regimen had not suffered that stupid interruption! Sadly, they have given up over a misconception.

Yes, fitness is hard earned and the idea of losing any of it is disheartening. But unless you stop exercising for years, it is never anywhere near as hard to get back to where you were as it was to get there the first time. Once your body has experienced a certain degree of adaptation to an exercise stimulus, returning to that degree of adaptation will always be easier in the future. In other words, you can always get it back.

If, for example, you were to spend a month on a deserted island lounging in a hammock, you might return to your workouts to find that your strength had declined a bit and that you were a little quicker to lose your breath. However, each post-vacation workout will be a huge step toward your previous fitness achievements, and you will probably be right back to your pre-vacation form within two weeks. Depending on how much punishment you put your body through during your downtime, getting back in the saddle could take more or less time, but I have never seen a situation in which someone required more than a few weeks to get back in the swing of things even after as much as a few months away.

Your results are never so fleeting as to vanish forever the first time a break is forced upon you. They are still yours if you want them and fear is not a good enough reason to stop wanting them.

# *Finding Some Help*

I am sad to say it, but the fitness industry is not a homogeneous landscape of impeccable knowledge and excellent value. It is composed largely of big corporate gyms that basically offer space and equipment for rent and small boot-camp-type gyms that sometimes seem to believe every workout should be a trip to the edge of insanity. Sprinkle on copious amounts of ridiculous marketing hype delivered by fitness models and what we have ended up with is a travesty. Training ranging from *out-of-this-world extraordinary* to *you-gotta-be-kidding-me terrible* can be found in both gym types.

As I mentioned earlier, you may find that you need someone to show you the ropes so you can get off to a good start without hurting yourself or wasting your time, and I generally think that's the way to go. That does not mean everyone will need or want long-term training, only that the vast majority of beginners would best be served by getting some professional help with their form.

There are plenty of amazing coaches and trainers out there, but throwing yourself blindly to the wolves is not advised. When you don't know what to look for, everything sounds good. If a trainer helps you lose ten pounds of fat, you might sing his praises even while he is beating your joints to a pulp, or having you squat heavy without addressing the lack of mobility in your hips, or spending five minutes teaching you how to do a complicated movement like the clean and jerk and then telling you to do a hundred reps for time, or... OK, I think you get the point.

So what are you supposed to do? Obviously, if your only option is to fully educate yourself on all this stuff, you won't really need a trainer. But if you are looking for a trainer, there are a few telltale signs that you have found someone who can guide you to your goals.

First, look for someone who walks the walk and talks the talk of this book. If he wants to prescribe cardio and starvation for fat loss, keep looking. If he wants to stuff you full of supplements, keep looking. If he wants to put you on a low-fat vegetarian diet, run as fast as you can.

Second, be sure to find someone who does not believe that exercise alone holds all the answers you seek. If she doesn't have a strong grasp of Paleo nutrition, keep looking.

Third, you must find someone who is passionate about what she does and has a high regard for the science behind her craft. Unfortunately, most of the trainers you will encounter chose this line of work solely because they love to work out. Since they can't work out all day, they decided to get into the fitness industry so they could at least spend a lot of time in the gym around other people who are working out. It's not enough.

A great trainer is someone who is driven to keep learning by reading the pertinent scientific literature and staying on top of the research. Every exceptional trainer I know follows an obnoxious amount of blogs and podcasts and has other resources where new information can be found and dissected. They all have mentors they can turn to when they get stumped by a new situation with a client. How do you find all this out about them? You ask. When you interview trainers, and interviewing is exactly what you should do, this is what you should ask them:

Ask how they came to be trainers. They should tell you a story that sounds a lot better than "I was driving by the gym and saw a Help Wanted sign, so I stopped. I was hired on the spot, and the rest is history. These have been the best four days of my life!"

Ask about their education, especially the stuff outside of school and certifications, like seminars and books. If someone is willing to spend his own money and time on becoming better at what he does, he probably loves what he does. If he is not interested in continuing his education, training is just a job. You want someone who wants to do this forever and keep improving.

Ask what they would do if you got stuck and your progress stalled. You should hear something about analysis here. They should be interested in taking a closer look at your diet, sleep patterns, stress, etc. If their answer is more exercise without addressing any other variables, keep looking.

Finally, ask them if you can talk to at least one of their clients. This might not always be possible because some trainers tend to attract a very private clientele, but most good trainers will be totally comfortable with introducing you to other clients and leaving you to talk to them privately. In fact, most good trainers would probably prefer this situation because it will mean an easy sell for them.

Actually, the best thing you can do to find a great trainer is to put your ear to the ground. Well, not literally, because that would just make you look like a nut job and you'd probably get stepped on, but you know what I mean. Good reputations are built by two types of trainers: those who are loved for their personalities and those who do excellent work. You want the latter. A good cheerleader may be able to get you started, but you need them to finish the job. Your friends and acquaintances may not know the difference, but if you ask everyone you know, you will eventually find someone who knows someone who can't shut up about her amazing trainer.

Spend a little time finding the right trainer and learn the basics. If you are tight on cash, strike out on your own after you have been properly educated, but at least grab a few sessions to learn the basic movement patterns from someone qualified to teach them. After that, throw in some of your own motivation, and the sky's the limit for you.

# CHAPTER 19

## it's never too late to get in the game

### Never Too Old!

If you are over thirty, this section is for you. If you are still in your twenties (or younger), I encourage you to follow along to gain a clearer picture of what might happen to you.

It is disheartening, and more than a little maddening, that the medical community has led most people to believe that aging means a slow and steady loss of vitality, a predictable rate of fat gain, and eventually the consistent addition of more pharmaceutical drugs to their daily pill-gobbling routine. If we all resign ourselves to being "normal," it seems that we are meant to lament every moment past our thirtieth birthday as another moment of not being as good as we were in our twenties. I will put this misguided nonsense to rest, but first I need to make sure that you are willing to listen to reason. I have actually been ferociously attacked for suggesting what I am about to suggest: If you think you are in pretty good shape *for your age*, it's time to think differently.

Getting older is not a valid excuse for getting fat, weak, and unhealthy. I'm sorry to state it so plainly, but it must be said. If you insist on clinging to this mind-set after reading this chapter, you need to put this book down and meditate on your situation for a while. Your ability to achieve the results you want are dependent on your ability to eat and exercise and live your life as if you believe your goals are within reach. Unfortunately, if you set those goals based on the mainstream perspective, you will sell yourself far short of the health and physical capacity you are truly capable of realizing.

Age often comes with one huge benefit over youth: The older you get, the more the desire to feel good outweighs the desire to look good. If you have grasped one of the major underlying themes of this book, you understand that the pursuit of peak health will actually lead to looking great, too, but maybe without all the self-torment that comes with purely aesthetic goals. If you are here to feel better, thank your lucky stars. Have faith in what I am laying down here, and you will be ecstatic with your results.

## Deb, Fifty-Three Years Old

Deb was almost fifty when we first met. To be honest, she had lived almost fifty years, but her body seemed much older. She was a nice woman with a warm smile, but there wasn't any vibrancy behind her eyes. She had the all too common look of a middle-aged American woman who had spent her adult life giving freely of herself to those she loved without ever stopping to consider her health or vitality. But Deb had one very important advantage over most women her age: she had not resigned herself to the sentence handed down to women by "common knowledge" regarding aging. She felt like bloody hell and she was fed up.

Deb owns a restaurant, and she couldn't work longer than six hours at that time before her aches and pains would relegate her to tears in her recliner. The stairs in her home were enough to sap her energy and force her to stop and catch her breath. She enjoyed working in the garden, but that was also becoming more difficult and less enjoyable. One day, Deb fell off a ladder in her yard and landed with her neck dangerously close to the open blades of a pair of pruning shears. Her family put their collective feet down and told her she was no longer allowed to work in the yard alone. She was frustrated and saddened by the loss of an activity that brought her joy, and all because her body seemed to be falling apart.

Deb was borderline diabetic with bursitis in her knees and hips. She had a duodenal bleeding ulcer and a heart flutter. She took meds for pain that her doctors said was caused by systemic inflammation (an extremely vague diagnosis, in my opinion, but what do I know?). She also had arthritis in her hip, but she was told that everyone her age has arthritic hips. On the cusp of fifty, she was taking five prescription drugs, and her doctor was adamant that she was doing great for her age. There was one year when Deb was on antibiotics more than she was off them.

"I knew I had to do something," Deb said. "I kept asking my doctor why it was always another pill or another physical therapy session, but I was still getting sicker and we weren't talking about the root of my problems. Why weren't we talking about what was causing me to get more and more sick?"

Like most people, Deb believed that pills should solve her problems, but they weren't. Eventually, her perspective began to change. "I realized I was going to have to figure this out on my own," she said, "and I thought, 'This is going to be really hard.' But it occurred to me that I didn't get that way overnight." Just as with Angela, the brilliance of someone able to see her situation with enough clarity to ask the right questions began to shine.

Deb was referred to me by her son Cooper, who also happens to be my friend, and arrived at my gym humbly asking for my help. Her situation was perfect for making huge changes. She was so miserable and frustrated that she has described her attitude by saying, "You couldn't do anything to me that was worse than where I was at that time." Not to make light of her situation, but she was the type of client who is every trainer's dream. She was willing to do *everything* I told her to do in *exactly* the way I told her to do it. No questions, no complaining, no deviating from the plan. This made Deb a semi-rare commodity in my world. Can you guess why? Yep, her *perspective* was right and she *wanted change more than she wanted any of the alternatives.* These are hard to come by if you are driven only to change the way you look with no consideration for improving your health. You might forget your desire to look good when faced with chocolate cake, but no food on earth will make you forget feeling as if you had one foot in the grave. Interestingly, many people still go for garbage foods, but not Deb. She saw her body as something worthwhile and she chose to save it.

Another point worth mentioning is that Deb surveyed the journey before she set out on it and knew it would be difficult, but she was not scared. Here again, we see the extraordinary person that is Deb. Fear really has no hold on someone with enough desire, and desire was something that Deb had in spades. When new people walk into my gym for their first assessment, the vast majority of them are stricken with terror. I am certainly not saying that this is a bad thing or an indication that they will fail; it is OK to be afraid. However, the absence of fear in someone with such a compromised body is often a sign that she truly wants what she came for. It is not very difficult to step outside your comfort zone if it means achieving a goal that is very important to you.

My role was roughly the same in Deb's journey as it was in Angela's. I didn't really do much except give Deb the information she was so desperately seeking. She brought a ravenous appetite for this information and a willingness to apply it with all the vigor of someone who really meant it when she said she wanted change. Change came quickly.

Here are Deb's before and after photos.

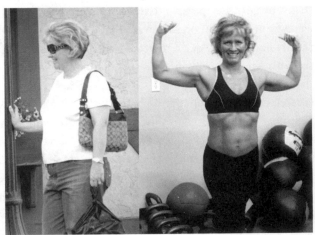

Notice how on the left she looks like a grandma and on the right she looks as if she should be wearing a cape flowing in the wind as she stands atop a pile of vanquished villains. She went from a size 22 at her biggest, to a size 0, and then to the ripped size 4 you see here. The amazing part is that Deb couldn't care less about these aesthetic changes. They are small (sweet) potatoes compared to everything else she has gained. In fact, when you ask Deb what she has accomplished since she found her new Paleo lifestyle, she usually forgets to include the appearance stuff. Ask that question of someone who starved himself into smaller pants, and all you will hear about is smaller pants. And the big pants are only on a short vacation, soon to return.

"I was totally unaware of my physical changes on the outside until people started asking me about my workout plan or what was in my shopping cart," Deb said. "I didn't understand why they were asking me, but then I realized that I must look as healthy as I feel. So many of my women friends commented on my looks and I would almost feel sad for them. If only they could feel the way I feel, they would forget all about how they look and jump into their new life with both feet!"

Deb was out with her five-year-old twin granddaughters one day when someone said, "Wow! You are in great shape for having twins!" Hilarious, but also thought-provoking. While there are certainly beautiful women at every age, you are probably in excellent health if people think you are at least a decade younger than your actual age. Starving yourself smaller does not result in a youthful glow.

I remember a conversation I had with Deb in which I told her that I didn't want to qualify her accomplishments with her age anymore. I didn't want to finish bragging about her by saying, "... which is great for a woman her age." She was already making excellent progress, but she still had a few self-imposed limitations she was having trouble getting over. "But Jason," she said, "I'm fifty years old!" I can still hear her pleading voice, and it makes me smile to know that she never really let herself believe what she was implying with those words.

Beginning with her physical capacity in the gym, here are some of the things Deb can do today:

Back Squat: 195 lbs.
Shoulder Press: 85 lbs.
Dead Lift: 265 lbs. (Tied for second place for all women in my gym.)
Bench Press: 117.5 lbs.
Weighted Chin-ups: 35 lbs. (*Yes, you read that correctly. Deb can do a chin-up with 35 pounds added to her body weight!*)
One-Mile Run: 8 min 45 s
1,000-Meter Row: 4 min 35 s

I have a video of Deb performing a strict pull-up after approximately eight months of training and Paleo nutrition. Many *young* women tend to assume that pull-ups are not possible, but Deb took the challenge at fifty.

Cooper once told her that she has undergone a huge personality change. He said she never used to smile or laugh or have any fun, and that all she ever said was no. "She wasn't really my mom before," Cooper said. "She was basically checked out. Now she is happy, full of energy, and adventurous."

Some of the adventures Deb has pursued in the last couple of years are paintball, bouldering and rock climbing, roller-skating, cycling, and ziplining. To be honest, I don't know very many people in their twenties who enjoy so many physically demanding activities.

Deb and her husband, Mike, have always had a good marriage, but now they share a fresh new level of intimacy and closeness that is "better than good." Deb said, "We are best friends, soul mates. We are deliriously happy." Grinning, she added, "Mike introduces me to people as his beautiful wife, and then he tells them about all my accomplishments in the gym. I let him go on for a while before I stop him."

Shall we stop right there? I can say without question that I would personally trade quite a lot for nothing more than the improved moods and increased energy Deb experienced, and I would fight tooth and nail to keep them, but a great relationship is immeasurable. However, this is not a good place for a bookmark because we have only just begun to share in Deb's joy over her new life.

Below is the list of improvements Deb refers to as "normal stuff":

◦ She sleeps like a rock, uninterrupted and solid.

◦ Her vitality has increased dramatically. "No more sleepwalking through life," she said. "As I became healthy, it was like I was coming out of a coma. The sky was bluer, the grass was greener, and the air was sweeter."

◦ Her skin has improved. "Most of my wrinkles that were supposedly associated with age are gone! No more nasty breakouts, either."

◦ No more kidney stones. "I had them for ten years," Deb said. "As soon as I started changing my diet and lifestyle, those little rocks started leaving one at a time. A couple of the bigger ones needed the help of a laser, but they are all gone now."

◦ No more mood swings.

◦ No more hot flashes. "Except when I work out," Deb told me with a laugh.

◦ Deb couldn't be on her feet for more than a few hours a day. "Now I can be on my feet all day and walk miles if I choose."

◦ The most astonishing change for me was the nearly complete reversal of Deb's menopause symptoms. Her monthly cycle has even returned. "Each month it shows up like clockwork," she said, "but with no cramps or PMS, which makes it a joy to be a healthy woman, not a curse. It's a big compliment from my body, as far as I am concerned, that it sees me as healthy enough to reproduce."

◦ Her hair is thick and shiny again, whereas it was unhealthy and thinning before Paleo.

◦ "I also had those wild black hairs that would pop out on my chin and neck," Deb said. "But they don't come back anymore."

◦ Her fingernails are strong again, so she doesn't wear fake nails anymore.

◦ "My eyelashes are back, and I don't feel the need to wear much makeup, if any."

▫ She is pain-free! "I remember sobbing for hours over the pain I felt. I am so grateful that it is all gone now." You can see true happiness on Deb's face when she talks about this one. Living with pain can suck the life out of anyone.

▫ By necessity, Deb used to know where the restroom was at all the places she frequented. Even sneezing might have caused her to lose control of her bladder. "At the risk of giving away too much here, I had several pelvic-floor issues—bladder, uterus, etc. I am happy to report that today they are in as good of shape as the rest of me!"

▫ She can breathe more easily. "I was a three-pack-per-day smoker years ago and I developed asthma and other respiratory issues," Deb said. "Things improved when I quit smoking, but I didn't regain my lung capacity until I got healthy."

▫ Her heart flutter is gone. "I had a flutter in one of my valves," she said. "It wasn't life-threatening, but my doctor was keeping an eye on it. It went away after about six months of Paleo and healthy exercise."

▫ Deb was borderline diabetic and now she does not even have any symptoms that could be precursors to the disease.

▫ Her blood pressure is 96/58, and her resting heart rate is 58. We tend to see numbers like these in athletes and kids, not fifty-three-year-old women.

▫ "Lastly, I learned how to take care of myself and take responsibility for my own choices," she said. "I am in the driver's seat of my own life now."

As you can see, this list of improvements is nothing short of amazing. Deb went from one of the most deconditioned people I have ever worked with to one of the most physically capable, and these claims are irrespective of age. What would you trade for this to be your list? When I hear stories like Deb's, I cannot help but think that there is simply not a junk food so flavorful, a workout so hard, or any comfort zone so cozy as to trump these benefits. What do you think?

# *Mike, Forty-Eight Years Old*

Now let's talk about Mike, Deb's husband, for a bit of the male point of view. No question about it, Mike is one of my favorite clients. Like Deb, he is a hard person to dislike.

Let me start by giving you a little trainer insight. I'm generalizing here, but men can sometimes be hard to motivate because they are often driven only by capacity goals. In other words, getting them to eat right or work on mobility can be like pulling teeth because they don't see how they're related to lifting enormous weights, or doing more pull-ups, or sprinting faster than the next guy, or whatever else might be today's measure of manliness. I was once guilty of these misperceptions myself, so I totally get it. But now that my own head is on right, it can be quite frustrating to try to make the average guy realize that he has to get healthier to reach his goals. Maybe Deb set a great example, but Mike made it easy on me.

When Mike came for his assessment he was in typical shape for his age. In other words, he was probably a heck of a lot more deconditioned than he thought he was. As we age, some of us men tend to hold on to the fantasy that we are still the superheroes we once believed ourselves to be. Our physical capacity may deteriorate, but it is not tested often enough over the years to cause any alarm.

I sent Mike out for a 200-meter run that first day, which is only halfway around a standard track. He had to walk to the finish, and was still huffing and puffing and drenched with sweat as if he had just run a marathon. Like Deb, Mike had been a smoker, and his lung capacity was significantly compromised.

We moved on to some bodyweight movements and light weights. Like many men, his mobility was pretty bad. He seemed to be tight everywhere, and as can be expected, his limited range of motion forced him into unsafe positions in some of the basic gym movements, like squatting and dead-lifting. I was sure we were in for a long road to fit and healthy, but Mike had other ideas. He fell in love with the process and made unbelievable strides.

The photos on the next page are from a ten-week contest we held in my gym, which Mike won. The photo on the left was taken and submitted to me on January 9, 2010. The photo on the right was taken and submitted to me on March 20, 2010.

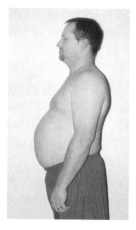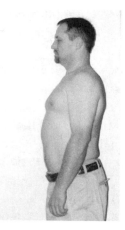

It is easy to see why Mike won. These results are astonishing! But losing his belly is just one benefit. Here are some of things Mike can do in the gym today:

Back Squat: 325 lbs.
Shoulder Press: 165 lbs.
Dead Lift: 340 lbs.
Bench Press: 215 lbs.
One-Mile Run: 7 min 11 s (Same guy who couldn't run 200 meters!)

Those are impressive numbers for anyone at any age, but if we buy into the hype, forty-eight-year-old men should not be capable of achieving these numbers at all. OK, so Mike was in bad shape and now he is in good shape, what of it? Well, there is more to the story.

Prior to Mike finding Paleo nutrition and getting on board with healthy, responsible exercise, he appeared to be walking down a scary path. Mike's daughter is a caregiver in a facility for Alzheimer's patients. One day she called Deb and said, "You have got to do something about my dad. I am convinced that he is in the beginning stages of Alzheimer's disease. I've had conversations with him and he can't remember anything I said. He can't remember where he put things; he is always losing his keys. He acts a lot like the people I work with, and he won't listen to me when I tell him he needs to see a doctor about this!" Deb also saw these symptoms in Mike, but it was especially alarming coming from someone who had firsthand experience with Alzheimer's patients. Fortunately, Paleo came to the rescue before an intervention was imposed on Mike by his family. Today, Mike is sharp as a tack, his brain working at full speed, and his loved ones are relieved. Needless to say, this one anecdote could provide reason enough to try Paleo. Talk about dodging a bullet!

Mike was also snoring heavily and suffering from sleep apnea. As you can imagine, it is hard to sleep next to someone who stops breathing periodically, and Deb was forced to move into their guest room to get a good night's sleep. Now that Mike is fit and healthy, the snoring and sleep apnea are gone and Deb has happily returned to her place at his side.

Just like Deb, Mike was forced to do battle with the stairs in their house several times a day, and it often seemed as if the stairs were winning. "I would only have to go up the stairs and I would be winded," he said. "We were actually thinking about selling the house because of those stairs." It is sad to think that these people I know and love were nearly forced out of their home because its floor plan was becoming an insurmountable obstacle in their day-to-day lives. Of course, now those stairs aren't given a second thought.

Those stairs were not the only thing challenging Mike's stamina. Mike is a printing press operator, and sometimes he needs to move quickly, but his deconditioned state was getting in the way. In printer speak he said, "If I had to run from my folder to my units, I would be out of breath and it would take me awhile to recover." Now Mike could spend the whole day doing those laps, if necessary.

Without going into too much detail, Mike had digestive issues that were problematic enough to warrant a trip to the doctor's office. He was referred to a specialist, who suggested pills (big surprise) and a colonoscopy. Mike's exact response was, "Doc, if you want to look up my ass you have got too much time on your hands!" I laughed until I nearly fell over when Mike told me this story. I am not suggesting that tests aren't useful diagnostics, and I am not condoning his decision to avoid them, but the point is that Mike decided to go at his problems differently. Paleo eventually took care of Mike's digestive issues.

To top it all off, Mike says that he was twenty-three years old and in the Marine Corps the last time he was as physically fit as he is today. He also cannot remember the last time he got sick. Even if we knew nothing about Mike's pre-Paleo condition, his current condition would be fantastic and enviable. When we throw in all the real-life benefits that have come to light for Mike, his story becomes an irrefutable cheer of "Paleo works!"

I know this all seems like a typical diet-and-exercise testimonial, and I said I would not do that, but the message I would really like to get across to the men is that you should not take any aspect of your health for granted. You are not "just getting old." You do not have to resign yourself to aches and pains and a dysfunctional body that refuses to do what you ask of it. The good news is that you can reclaim your body by eating steaks and engaging in manly activities like lifting heavy things, sweating, and talking trash with the guys. I am a man and I am as testosterone ridden as any, so please don't lie to me and say that you are completely willing to let go of your desire to express your manliness. Come back out and play!

## Debbie, Fifty-Seven Years Old

Debbie, not to be confused with Deb, is another amazing woman whom it has been my pleasure to know. She is fifty-seven, but her body has no concept of time. To be honest, Debbie was never very big. Her "before" and "after" pictures are great, but not showstopping.

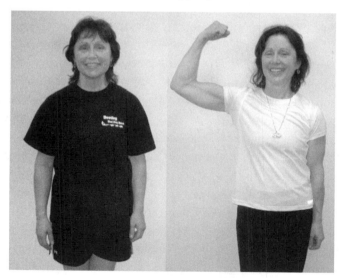

The real reason I want to tell you about Debbie is to put another nail in the coffin of the "you are just getting old" fallacy. Some of you are reading these stories and thinking, "Well, that is just fine for those gifted individuals, but I am just a regular person, and I really am getting old!" I'm hoping that if I give you enough examples, complete with all the trials these folks faced to get where they are, maybe you will see yourself in one of them and take back your health.

Debbie is an excellent example of how an active lifestyle can still allow aging to creep in if mainstream health and nutrition advice is still a big part of the picture. She is a competitive sled dog racer. She runs a four-dog team and was the Pacific Northwest champion in the 2007-08 and 2008-09 seasons. She has since become interested in Canadian races, which has taken her out of the running in the Northwest. There are no gender or age classes in dog sledding, which means that Debbie races against women and men sometimes half her age in this physically demanding sport. Interestingly, she has conveyed to me that many of her competitors seem to think the sport is all about the dogs, neglecting their own health and fitness. Debbie held this view herself until her body began to slow her down.

Even though she was never very heavy, Debbie went on many diets in the past in pursuit of fat loss. "Years ago I did the low-fat thing," she said. "I never stuck to any one diet for very long, except that for years I ate very little meat. In fact, when I first found your gym I was only eating fish and chicken. I just thought it was better for me."

When I asked her what brought her to me, she replied, "I was starting to feel old. Getting up in the morning, my back hurt and my energy level was depleted. That just wasn't working for me."

Like most people, Debbie had to force herself out of her comfort zone. "Honestly," she said, "when I looked at your Web site I was scared. I didn't want to embarrass myself." How many people stop right there? There is no way to know for sure, but I am positive the percentages are high. Comfort zones are usually quite comfy, and leaving them requires courage. Debbie decided that her desire to feel better far outweighed the risk of looking silly in front of complete strangers.

Debbie started eating Paleo and working out with me in May 2010 and noticed big changes very quickly. Before 2007, Debbie raced with a team of dogs that weren't very fast, and racing wasn't very physically demanding for her. In 2007 she got a new team. Her new dogs were much faster, and Debbie was suddenly working hard to keep up and stay on the sled. "In the next race season after finding Paleo and proper exercise," she said, "one of the first things I noticed was that I had a lot more confidence in my ability to navigate my sled around technical courses. Those previous couple of years I was crashing and burning."

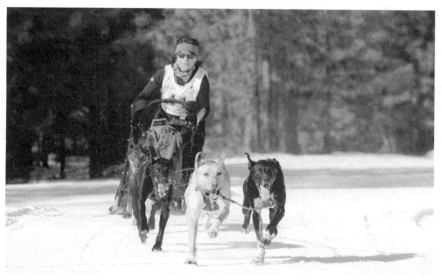

*Here is Debbie doing what she loves to do*

I understand, of course, that you are probably not a sled dog racer. In fact, you may not compete in any sports at all, and that is totally fine, provided that's your preference. In other words, not playing a sport because you choose not to is perfectly fine, but not playing a sport because your body refuses to cooperate is unacceptable. I suppose I am imposing my own values on you here, but I just don't believe you should let your body make such decisions for you. I am guessing that if you have read this far you agree.

Debbie actually discovered many benefits outside of her sport, as well. Working around her country home is much easier for her now. She explained, "I am always lifting things and building things and moving things around. All of it is easier now, and that was my main goal." How much easier? We can get a good idea by looking at what she can do in the gym:

Back Squat: 150 lbs.
Shoulder Press: 70 lbs.
Dead Lift: 205 lbs.
Bench Press: 95 lbs.
One-Mile Run: 8 min 35 s
500-Meter Row: 2 min 8 s
Debbie can also perform two or three strict pull-ups in a row.

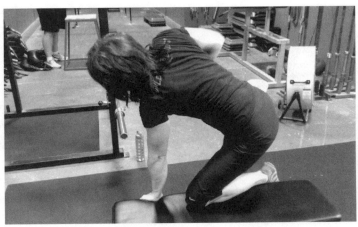

*Does this look like a fifty-seven-year-old woman?*

"I don't care if I ever set a record lifting heavy weights," Debbie said. "My goal was to be stronger in my everyday life." After reviewing those numbers, I think it is safe to say that Debbie is well equipped to handle most anything that needs doing around her house. As with Mike and Deb, Debbie's story would stand on its own if we stopped right here, but it gets better.

"I used to take a medication for migraines," Debbie said. "But when I went in for my annual checkup last year my doctor asked me if I needed a refill, and I realized I had not taken it in months." Before Paleo and proper exercise, she suffered a migraine approximately once a month, and her doctors thought there was an underlying hormonal cause. Debbie may never know for sure what caused her migraines, but they are gone.

Menopause affects women in a different ways, and it made Debbie irritable. I can't speak from experience on this one, but it must be a huge relief to dodge a symptom that makes you grumpy. "I am a way nicer person now," Debbie said, laughing.

I asked Debbie if she has better digestion now and she said, "Oh, absolutely! I didn't realize how bad I felt because of what I was eating until I started Paleo."

Sugar addiction was a problem for Debbie too. "Sugar was big for me," she said. "And that may have come from the low-fat era. Sugar was OK as long as you avoided fat." We shared a good laugh about this. Of course, it is easy for us to be amused now that we both know better, but we are definitely the minority in a world that vilifies fat much more than sugar. Getting serious again, Debbie said, "Every once in a while I will be tempted by sugar, but especially if there are grains involved, like cake, it just makes me sick." The disgusted look on her face when she said this told me she meant it.

Of all the positive changes Debbie has experienced, the thing that struck the biggest chord with me was hearing her say, "I'm out there doing the things I want to do and I never get hurt. I really forget how old I am." I think those two sentences sum it all up nicely. Translation: "I'm truly living, not merely existing."

## Tim, Sixty-One Years Old

Tim is another great example demonstrating that age should be decisively removed from our list of valid excuses to get healthy and fit. Tim is sixty-one, he came to me when he was sixty, and he is a pleasure to train. He found the right perspective before he sought my assistance, so all he needed from me were the details.

The people who walk into my gym and proceed to accomplish amazing things very quickly always have two things in common: they knew what they wanted and they came equipped with the motivation to get it. Tim is one of these people.

In his twenties and thirties Tim was in great shape. He worked hard and played hard. But Tim owns a successful flooring store, and like many business owners, he eventually found himself doing more managerial duties and moving around less. Jump ahead thirty years, and his days of excellent physical conditioning had slipped away.

Installing flooring can be tough on the body, and Tim ended up with a low-back injury in his late thirties that has been an intermittent problem ever since. "It would come and go," he said. "If I picked up something wrong it would give me trouble. I just don't think those muscles back there were strong enough."

Tim is a hunter and a golfer and in the couple of years prior to his sixtieth birthday his body was not keeping up with his desire to avidly pursue these activities. It's one thing to lose interest in something, or have new interests nudge out old ones, but losing your ability to do the things you love for no better reason than that your body is slowly applying the brakes is frustrating. This is the position Tim found himself in. His body had not told him to stop hunting and golfing yet, but it was beginning to protest.

"I couldn't golf two days in a row," Tim said. "If I golfed one day, either my back was out the next day or I was just too sore to go again." Being an avid golfer in the Northwest United States means squeezing rounds in when the weather permits. In the spring and fall, two nice days in a row can be hard to come by, so missing the opportunity to golf two beautiful days in a row because of a body that will not cooperate can be maddening.

Tim's situation was the same on hunting trips. Hunting elk with a bow requires hiking for miles in treacherous terrain. After two hunts a day, a long one in the morning and a shorter one in the evening, Tim usually racked up seven to ten miles a day. "Sometimes one day's hunt would leave me too tired to hunt the next day," he said. "I had pain in my shoulders and knees, and I didn't feel very sure-footed." It goes without saying that hunting trips are short adventures, not extended or ever-present opportunities. Obviously it is more fun to hunt everyday. Can you imagine planning a trip, spending the money to make it happen, and then sitting around camp half the time because your body objected to your original plans? Saying "I'm just getting old" offers little comfort while you watch the things you love slip through your fingers.

The summer before Tim came to me, his back went out worse than it ever had. "Usually within a few days it would straighten out a bit," he said. "But this time it hurt for weeks." He saw a chiropractor for a while, but it became apparent to him that his back problems would always return if he didn't take control and get in better shape.

Through the combination of turning sixty and his aches and pains, Tim was ready for change. "I didn't want to be shaky or walk like an old man," he said. "I wanted to get the spring back in my step. I wanted to be able to jump up into the back of my truck whenever I needed to. I wanted to be able to do all the things I used to do." Tim also wanted better stress management. The downturn in the economy in 2008 was tough on everyone, especially those of us who own businesses, and Tim was right there with the rest of us. He said, "I kind of felt like being in shape would allow me to handle stress better too."

As luck would have it, Tim already had the one advantage that I am trying to give you at this very moment. "My hunting partner, Frank, is seventy-three, and he could walk off and leave me behind on the hills," Tim told me with a grin. This was a big motivator for Tim. When we first met, I asked him why he wanted to get in shape. He chuckled and said, "I'm tired of my hunting partner laughing at me whenever I try to get over a fence."

Fortunately for Tim, Frank is an excellent example of fitness and vitality, despite being more than a decade Tim's senior. I am not sure that Tim would ever have made excuses, but it is difficult to hold on to an excuse when someone close to you puts the lie to it on a regular basis, and it is especially difficult when that person has more of a right to the excuse than you do.

However it happened, Tim is a rare exception to the norm because he does not buy into the view that aging should mean watching your body fall apart. "If you think you are getting old, you feel old, and all you want to talk about is your aches and pains. I don't think you have to go that way. I knew I could get my body back in shape and get back to doing the things I wanted to do." Listening to Tim say those things was an awesome experience for a trainer. Once again, I received further proof that perspective is everything.

Tim is a regular guy who had no advantage over anyone else except for his exceptional perspective. When the world offered him the standard aging excuse, he turned it down instead of owning it and ardently selling it to all who would listen, as is customary. Big things happen when a person's perspective is right. "I knew that I could get in shape and help myself," Tim said. "But I didn't know I would be able to do the things I can do now."

Tim arrived at my gym with all his aches and pains, out of shape, but ready to get to work. The picture below shows his condition at that time. With him is his lovely wife, Elane, who is another fantastic Paleo success story.

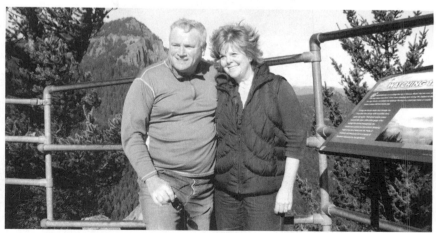

*Tim, before adopting a Paleo lifestyle, and his beautiful wife Elane*

While it is true that Tim looks great (Elane says he has become a "chick magnet"), and it is obvious just by looking that he is healthier now, his primary reasons for seeking change were about feeling and performing better. You can decide for yourself if you think Tim has achieved exceptional physical capacity. Here are a few of his accomplishments:

Back Squat: 235 lbs.
Dead Lift: 275 lbs.
Bench Press: 175 lbs.
Shoulder Press: 135 lbs.
Plank Hold: 3 min 3 s
500-meter Row: 1 min 40 s

Again, here we see numbers that indicate well-rounded physical capacity for any age. When I brag about Tim's abilities in the gym I do not have to mention his age at all. While the vast majority of people his age are either married to their limitations or accomplishing things that are "good for their age," Tim is doing things that are good for any age.

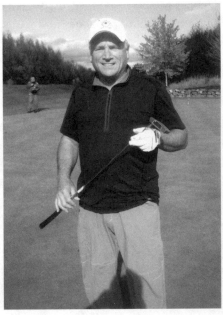

*Tim today*

What level of value do you think Tim places on his health and physical capacity now that he has made these amazing strides? He had to make room in his life for change, he had to get out of his comfort zone, and he worked his butt off, but do you think it was worth it? Do you think it would be worth it to him if he had to do ten times as much work to get these same results? I know what he would say, but what do you think?

## Elane, Sixty-Two Years Old

I have one more excellent example of age defiance for you that I just can't leave out. Elane is Tim's wife, and she is every trainer's dream client. Even though she is the oldest of the five people whose stories I have shared with you, she was not particularly miserable when she found me—she just wanted to get through life with a little more ease. She has eight grandkids that were beginning to outpace her, and she wanted to regain some of her youthful vigor so she wouldn't miss out on all the fun. Here is how Elane looked when Tim convinced her to come see me:

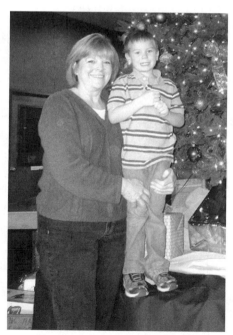

*Elane, pre-Paleo, with her grandson, Hayden*

Even though changing her appearance was not a primary motivation for Elane, she had been there in the past. In her thirties she began to attract some excess fat, and, as it does, it made her a little insecure about the way she looked. After three kids, her body was not cooperating the way it used to, and she wanted to do something about it.

It seemed obvious to her at the time that calories and saturated fat must be to blame for her weight gain, so Elane did what most people do and began jogging and joined popular weight-loss programs based on caloric restriction. Eventually, jogging morphed into cardio on treadmills and stair climbers at a gym, sprinkled with a bit of resistance training on machines. Unfortunately, none of it worked. "I would do diets and lose weight," she said, "and then realize that I couldn't eat that way for the rest of my life. As soon as I went back to eating the same old way I always had, I would gain it all back, but I just didn't want to be hungry all the time."

As frustrating as these failures were, nobody was offering any radically different options, so the cycle kept repeating itself. Elane said, "I would go on those diets and lose some weight, gain it all back, and then try something new. I even remember trying to see how long I could go in a day without eating and then try to only eat a little bit. I didn't feel good on any of the diets, and I was hard to be around because I was irritable." She is describing what is known as *dieting* to most people, and it is hell to be in. Whatever Elane did to try to lose weight would always make her feel worse. "I would lose weight," she said. "But there was a price to pay. I wasn't enjoying life." It is hard to justify paying anything at all for temporary results.

Shortly after I began working with Tim, he suggested that Elane give me a call. She did, we met, I instantly liked her, but she was terrified of me. Change is scary, and I can sometimes be all business, but she wanted results more than she wanted to stay in her comfort zone. We agreed to work together and got on it right away.

In the beginning, Elane made the common mistake of putting a Paleo spin on all of her favorite foods instead of truly changing the way she was eating. "I ate Paleo muffins, Paleo breads, Paleo smoothies, and I didn't see any results." It makes me sad that this happens to so many people, but they can hardly be blamed when cookbooks and recipe blogs abound perpetuating the notion that SAD foods can be shoehorned into the Paleo mold. Don't fall for it!

Sometime around her three-month mark, though, Elane got serious, and change came quickly. Today, her vitality has returned, she has more energy, and as an added bonus she now looks like this:

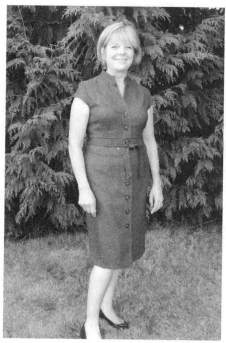

*Elane today*

Where once she would sit and watch her grandkids in the park, now El-ane plays with them as if she were a kid, too. I don't know about you, but I haven't seen many sixty-year-old women running and jumping and sliding and rolling around on the playground at my local park. People half Elane's age are usually bench-sitting spectators. Not Elane. "Bike rides, ice skating, swimming—I can do it all with them. And I don't freak out anymore when I have to put on a swimsuit," she said with a giggle.

Elane also used to be tuckered out after cleaning her house, but "now it's easy," she said. "I just do my chores and I still have the rest of my day." How nice not to have an entire day disappear after scrubbing a floor—household responsibilities should not require recovery time.

Remember, Elane did not start eating a Paleo diet and exercising accord-ing to the methods in this book until she was sixty-one. The majority of people her age have resigned themselves to their status quo. But Elane has accomplished some amazing feats. She said, "I never thought I would be able to run 400 meters in a workout without stopping to rest." Now she sometimes runs 400 meters three or four times in a one-hour training session. And look what she can do with a barbell:

Dead Lift: 145 lbs.
Shoulder Press: 55 lbs.
Bench Press: 75 lbs.
Box Squat: 100 lbs.

Those numbers are impressive for any woman, regardless of age, and Elane is still getting stronger all the time. In fact, there is a good chance that all of these numbers will have improved by the time you opened this book. Elane started later in life than all the people I've mentioned, but it didn't matter. Her accomplishments are equally amazing and worthwhile, and she wouldn't trade them for the world. I can't wait to see where she goes next.

# You Can Too!

If I have done my job well, Deb, Mike, Debbie, Tim, and Elane have helped you to understand that even defining aging as a minor inconvenience gives it power it doesn't deserve. These five remarkable individuals are remarkable only because of their perspective and their motivation. They took control of their health and fitness instead of hiding behind excuses. None of them have superpowers, none are genetically gifted, and all were considered "normal" by mainstream standards. If I had shared only one success story with you, you might think the person was a unique specimen with an unfair genetic advantage, but it's hard to refute success when five completely different people achieved it using the same methods. If these people achieved anything health- or fitness-wise that you desire, it is only because they made a decision that you are capable of making and then achieved things that you are capable of achieving.

You are the architect of your limitations. Too much time spent convincing yourself of what you can't do will set those limitations in stone. Instead, why not let your body tell you what it can do? Please do not misunderstand, running down to your nearest gym, completely deconditioned, and trying to see how much weight you can back squat for a 1 repetition maximum will likely get you hurt. But educating yourself, eating the way your body longs for you to eat, and advancing your physical capacity slowly and responsibly will take you to places you never thought you could go. As I have said before, nobody can tell you what you should value in your life, but hiding behind age or perceived physical restrictions is pointless. Taking a pill for every added devolvement of your health is even more pointless. You do not have to swallow the conventional "wisdom" (keyword: "conventional") about how good you should feel, about how you should expect your body to function. Do you want a body that works for you, or a body that is a burden? What you do now will decide. The choice is yours.

# EPILOGUE

Since you've made it this far, your perspective on health, and thereby fitness, should be forever changed. As I have said repeatedly throughout this book, perspective is everything. Seeing health and fitness for what they truly are will clear the path ahead of you, allowing you an unobstructed trek from here to your goals. Now it is time to apply what you know. Now comes the doing.

Get in the game. Don't delay. Start with baby steps if you like, but you don't have any valid reasons for not starting immediately, unless you've somehow decided, since the end of the previous paragraph, that your health and fitness aren't worth your time and effort, that you'd rather keep spending your time and energy on other aspects of your life. But I don't believe that's the case.

You now know that health is the only true path to sustainable aesthetic results. Therefore, it's time to ditch your scale, get out from under your own hypercritical eye in the mirror, and begin to eat and move like a real human being. The only other option is to stay where you are, which is totally fine as long as you don't claim to want better for yourself. Ignorance was a valid excuse before today, but now you have the honest, unadulterated answers to that nagging question: How do I get a healthy, fit body that looks great? What you do with those answers is up to you. But, now that the mystery is removed, you really have only two options: to act or not to act.

Will it be easy to turn the way you treat your body on its head? No, and I would never say so, but it doesn't have to be as hard as most people make it. In as little as a month from right now you could find yourself in a place where Paleo nutrition and fitness are the norm, where feeling good every day is expected, and where you love yourself enough to avoid physical and psychological pitfalls without even thinking about it.

So what will you do? Will you carry on as always or will you change your life in amazing ways? You have the tools. The decision is yours.

Go forth and be awesome.

# Recommended Reading

*Everyday Paleo* and *Everyday Paleo Family Cookbook,* by Sarah Fragoso

*The Paleo Solution,* by Robb Wolf

*The Primal Blueprint,* by Mark Sisson

*It Starts with Food,* by Dallas and Melissa Hartwig

*The Protein Power Lifeplan,* by Dr. Michael R. Eades and Dr. Mary Dan Eades

*Lights Out: Sleep, Sugar, and Survival,* by T.S. Wiley and Bent Formby

*Good Calories, Bad Calories,* by Gary Taubes

*The Vegetarian Myth,* by Lierre Keith

*Paleo Slow Cooking,* by Chrissy Gower

*The Great Cholesterol Con,* by Dr. Malcolm Kendrick